AF565089

Evaluation of Quality of Care in Psychiatry

Proceedings of a Symposium Held at the Queen Street Mental Health Centre Toronto, Canada 1979

PERGAMON TITLES OF RELATED INTEREST

BOOKS

R. CATALANO Health, Behavior and the Community: An Ecological Perspective

W. S. DAVIDSON, J. R. KOCH, R. G. LEWIS, M. D. WRESINSKI Evaluation Strategies in Criminal Justice

J. A. MORELL Program Evaluation in Social Research

L. C. SOBELL, M. B. SOBELL, E. WARD Evaluating Alcohol and Drug Abuse Treatment Effectiveness: Recent Advances

D. N. WEISSTUB Law and Psychiatry, 1st Symposium

D. N. WEISSTUB Law and Psychiatry, 2nd Symposium

D. N. WEISSTUB Law and Psychiatry in the Canadian Context (in press)

JOURNALS

Evaluation and Program Planning

International Journal of Law and Psychiatry

Journal of Psychiatric Treatment and Evaluation

Evaluation of Quality of Care in Psychiatry

Edited by:

A. G. Awad, M.B., B. Ch., Ph.D., F.R.C.P.(C)
Associate Professor, Department of Psychiatry
University of Toronto

H. B. Durost, M.D., F.R.C.P.(C), F.R.C.Psych.
Professor, Department of Psychiatry
University of Toronto

W. O. McCormick, M.A., M.B., F.R.C.P., F.R.C.P.(C), F.R.C.Psych.
Associate Professor, Department of Psychiatry
University of Toronto

Pergamon Press

Toronto • Oxford • New York • Sydney • Paris • Frankfurt

Pergamon Press Offices:

Canada	Pergamon of Canada, Suite 104, 150 Consumers Road, Willowdale, Ontario, Canada M2J 1P9
U.K.	Pergamon Press Ltd., Headington Hill Hall, Oxford 0X3 0BW, England
U.S.A.	Pergamon Press Inc., Maxwell House, Fairview Park, Elmsford, New York, 10523, U.S.A.
Australia	Pergamon Press (Aust.) Pty. Ltd., P.O. Box 544, Potts Point, N.S.W. 2011, Australia
France	Pergamon Press SARL, 24 rue des Ecoles, 75240 Paris, Cedex 05, France
Federal Republic of Germany	Pergamon Press GmbH, Hammerweg 6, Postfach 1305, 6242 Kronberg-Taunus, Federal Republic of Germany

Copyright © 1980 Pergamon of Canada Ltd.

Canadian Cataloguing in Publication Data

Main entry under title:

Evaluation of quality of care in psychiatry

"Proceedings of a symposium held at the Queen Street Mental Health Centre, Toronto, Canada, 1979."
Includes index.
ISBN 0-08-025364-4

1. Mental health services — Evaluation — Congresses.
2. Psychiatry — Methodology — Congresses.
I. Awad, Awad G., 1934- II. Durost, H.B., 1925- III. McCormick, William O., 1929-
RC437.5.E92 362.2'1 C80-094280-9

All Rights Reserved. No part of this publication may be reproduced, stored in a retrieval system or transmitted in any form or by any means: electronic, electrostatic, magnetic tape, mechanical, photocopying, recording or otherwise, without permission in writing from the copyright holders.

In order to make this volume available as economically and as rapidly as possible the authors' typescripts have been reproduced in their original forms. This method unfortunately has its typographical limitations but it is hoped that they in no way distract the reader.

Printed in Canada

Contents

Foreword vii

Acknowledgements ix

Contributors xi

Introduction xiii

Abbreviations xv

Quality Assurance in Health Care *W.R. Fifer* 1

Discussion *W.M. Goldberg* 13

Ten Assumptions Which Cripple Psychiatrists' Participation in Quality Assurance *A. Richman* 19

Discussion *M.G.G. Thompson* 33

Evaluation of Patient Care and Hospital Accreditation *H.B. Durost* 41

Peer Review and the Use of Psychotropic Drugs *R. Dorsey* 49

Discussion *A.G. Awad* 77

Peer Review of Outpatient Psychological Services *G. Stricker* 81

Discussion *B. Willer* 91

Panel and General Discussion *Moderator – F.H. Lowy* 97

Concluding Remarks *J.C.A. Sibley* 113

Index 121

Foreword

This Symposium on Quality of Care in Psychiatry was opened by the Honorable Dennis Timbrell, Minister of Health for Ontario on June 22nd, 1979.

It marks the first in a series of annual symposia on topics of importance in psychiatric hospital practice; the symposia were instituted in recognition of complete rebuilding of Queen Street Mental Health Centre, Toronto, completed in early 1979.

Acknowledgements

We wish to acknowledge the support of the Ministry of Health, Ontario as well as the Administrator, Queen Street Mental Health Centre, (Q.S.M.H.C.) Toronto: Mr. M. J. Fisher.

We thank Mrs. C. Zboril, Mrs. H. Beetham and Mrs. N. Forbes for their valuable secretarial help and Mrs. P. Ohlendorf for excellent editorial assistance.

We are grateful to Dr. F. H. Lowy, Professor and Chairman, Department of Psychiatry, University of Toronto, for his support and encouragement.

The Symposium, whose proceedings are published in this book, was made possible by generous support from:

THE PHYSICIAN SERVICES' INCORPORATED FOUNDATION,

THE ROYAL COLLEGE OF PHYSICIANS AND SURGEONS OF CANADA,

WYETH LIMITED, CANADA.

ORGANIZING COMMITTEE

A. G. Awad
H. B. Durost
W. O. McCormick

Contributors

A. G. AWAD, M. B.,
Chief, Southwestern Service, Q.S.M.H.C., Associate Professor, Co-ordinator of Psychopharmacology, Department of Psychiatry, University of Toronto

RICHARD DORSEY, M.D.,
Chief of Psychiatry, Otto C. Epp Memorial Hospital, Cincinnati, Ohio; Former Field Consultant to A.P.A. Task Force on Peer Review; Chairman of A.P.A. Task Force on Psychopharmacological Criteria Development

HENRY B. DUROST, M. D.,
Professor, Department of Psychiatry, University of Toronto, Medical Director, Q.S.M.H.C.; Surveyor for the Canadian Council on Hospital Accreditation

WILLIAM R. FIFER, M. D.,
Senior Investigator, Health Services Research Centre, Professor of Medicine and Public Health, University of Minneapolis, Minnesota; Consultant to the Joint Commission of Accreditation of Hospitals

Wm. M. GOLDBERG, M. D.,
Chief of Medicine, St. Joseph's Hospital, Hamilton, Clinical Professor, McMaster University, Hamilton; Ontario

F. H. LOWY, M. D.,
Professor and Chairman, Department of Psychiatry, University of Toronto; Psychiatrist-in-Chief, Clarke Institute of Psychiatry, Toronto, Ontario

W. O. McCORMICK, M.A., M.B.,
Associate Professor, Co-ordinator of Continuing Education, Department of Psychiatry, University of Toronto; Director of Education, Q.S.M.H.C., Toronto, Ontario

CONTRIBUTORS

ALEX RICHMAN, M.D.,
National Health Scientist, Professor of Psychiatry and Preventive Medicine, Director, Training and Research Unit in Psychiatric Epidemiology, Dalhousie University, and the Abbie Lane Memorial Hospital, Halifax, Nova Scotia

JOHN C. A. SIBLEY, M.D.,
Professor, Department of Medicine and Clinical Epidemiology and Biostatistics, Associate Dean (Education), McMaster University, Hamilton, Ontario

GEORGE STRICKER, Ph.D.,
Professor and Associate Dean, Institute of Advanced Psychological Studies, Adelphi University, Garden City, New York; Chairman, National Advisory Panel, CHAMPUS/American Psychological Association Peer Review Project

M. G. G. THOMPSON, M.D.,
Associate Professor, Department of Psychiatry, University of Toronto; Executive Director, Chief of Staff, West End Creche, Child and Family Clinic, Toronto, Ontario

BARRY WILLER, Ph.D.,
Assistant Professor, Division of Community Psychiatry, New York State University at Buffalo, New York

Introduction

The choice of the topic of Evaluation of Quality of Care in Psychiatry for a symposium in 1979 reflects the wide interest and importance of the subject at this time in the development of psychiatry. In Canada the national and provincial Psychiatric Associations have had committees actively considering the best approach to quality of care review. The possibility that specialists may have to re-certify at specific time intervals has been discussed, although no mandatory re-certification or proof of continuing medical education was required by the Royal College of Physicians and Surgeons of Canada or by the Canadian Psychiatric Association when this symposium was held.

If the reader picks up this book believing that it will be a "How to Do It" guide to quality of care evaluation in psychiatry he will be disappointed. The value of the contributions from those who have already been deeply involved in the implementation of programs of evaluation is as much the experience of difficulties as the reporting of smooth success. Papers are included from United States contributors with experience in established evaluation programs; in addition there are papers from Canada where, as in Britain and other countries, evaluation programs are still at the stages of discussion and development. As pointed out by Dr. Barry Willer, the appropriate method of care evaluation depends on the particular health care delivery system. The systems in Canada, Britain and some other English-speaking countries differ greatly from the United States in the degree of government involvement. The contributions of Dr. Willer and Dr. Richman are of particular interest, being based on experience in both the United States and Canada.

Professional people have, by the nature of their professions, a great deal of independence of action. If reviews are to succeed they have to be acceptable to a large majority of the profession being reviewed. In psychiatry-perhaps even more so than other branches of medicine-there are considerable divergences of view about ideal treatment in a given situation. Review procedures must not be rigid. It was illustrated in Dr. Dorsey's presentation about drug treatment that the standards, to be acceptable to a majority of psychiatrists, had to represent general standards of acceptable practice, rather than ideals as they might be enunciated by a psychopharmacology expert.

One approach to improvement of quality of care has been to encourage-almost to the point of compulsion-attendance at continuing medical education. It cannot be assumed that this will enhance the quality of care unless altered treatment behavior can be demonstrated after the educational experiences. Anecdotal accounts have been heard both from the United States and from Britain about the effect of having to document continuing medical education attendance. From both countries we hear of doctors who sign up for educational sessions in order to establish the necessary number of credit hours and exercise their independence of action by sleeping through most of the sessions.

Quality of care evaluation has been described as a multi-million dollar "industry". It is hoped that these contributions will improve the quality of the "product" being bought with these dollars.

Toronto, Canada,

January 1980.

A. G. Awad
H. B. Durost
W. O. McCormick
Editors

Abbreviations

ACPF	Accreditation Council for Psychiatric Facilities
AMA	American Medical Association
CCHA	Canadian Council on Hospital Accreditation
CHAMPUS	Civilian Health and Medical Program for the Uniform Services
CMA	Canadian Medical Association
CME	Continuing Medical Education
CPA	Canadian Psychiatric Association
DHEW	Department of Health, Education and Welfare
JCAH	Joint Commission on Accreditation of Hospitals
LOS	Length of Stay
PATS	Psychiatric Audit Team Seminars
PSRO	Professional Standards Review Organizations
QSMHC	Queen Street Mental Health Centre
SCOPCE	Select Committee on Psychiatric Care Evaluation
USGPO	United States General Printing Office
VA	Veteran Administration

Quality Assurance in Health Care

William R. Fifer, M.D.

What is Quality?

The first problem one encounters in any attempt to assess or assure quality in health care services is how to define "quality." While Webster (1) defines "quality" as "degree of excellence" and "quality control" as "an aggregate of activities (as design analysis and statistical sampling with inspection for defects) designed to ensure adequate quality in manufactured products," others have argued that the concept is so elusive that it defies measurement. Robert Pirsig (2) reflected upon the concept as follows:

> Quality . . . you know what it is, yet you don't know what it is. But that's self-contradictory. But some things *are* better than others, that is, they have more quality. But when you try to say what quality is, apart from the things that have it, it all goes *poof*! There's nothing to talk about. But if you can't say what quality is, how do you know what it is, or how do you know that it even exists? If no one knows what it is, then for all practical purposes it doesn't exist at all. But for all practical purposes it really *does* exist. What else are the grades based on? Why else would people pay fortunes for some things and throw others in the trash pile? Obviously some things are better than others . . . but what's the "betterness"? . . . So round and round you go, spinning mental wheels and nowhere finding any place to get traction. What the hell is quality? What *is* it?

In order to get on with the task of discussing quality assurance in health care, we have elected to define "quality" as "the degree of adherence to a standard (or standards)." This operational definition assumes that if one is in possession of standards, and is capable of measuring the degree of adherence to such standards, one will produce an objective and reliable measurement of quality.

Measuring the quality of manufactured goods is relatively straightforward; the public expects quality assurance methods and quality control procedures to be applied to automobiles or television sets. A physician would be horrified to learn that the tetracycline capsule he prescribes is not backed up by systematic determinations of potency, purity, and effectiveness; he has come to expect it and his expectations are reinforced by federal regulations to protect both him and his patients.

Similarly, we expect quality controls to apply to services and the arts, despite the difficulty of deciding what a "good" haircut or violin concerto is. This difficulty led to the concept of peer evaluation or "peer review," which proceeds from the premise that only an equal (peer) could possibly judge the quality of an erudite or complex performance such as conducting a symphony, flying an airplane, or removing a diseased uterus. The public has come to expect quality control in the airline industry, ranging from ongoing aircraft inspection and maintenance to periodic evaluation of flight crew performance.

It is somewhat surprising that measurement-oriented professions like the health sciences, which routinely expect formal quality control in services they use (such as the clinical laboratory), should have delayed so long a systematic attempt to evaluate the quality of the health care transaction. Indeed, until very recently peer review was the only assurance of quality offered, probably because the health care encounter was viewed as such a complex interaction of erudition, judgement, and technical skill that only a peer could understand it much less evaluate it.

In a simpler day, peer review was an adequate mechanism despite its shortcomings (subjectivity, randomness, lack of reproducibility, etc.), because no real accountability pressure existed. Today, faced with an ever-expanding legal doctrine of professional and institutional liability, "quality control" in health care services takes on new importance. Experts are no longer immune from challenges of their expertise. Public accountability for both the cost and quality of medical care has grown in proportion to the growth of their party payment, especially that reimbursed by public funds (Medicare and Medicaid). Objective methods of review and evaluation of health care services have been mandated by U.S. Federal Law (PL92-603) and are required by professional organizations such as the Joint Commission on Accreditation of Hospitals (JCAH) as a condition of accreditation of health care facilities and programs.

As the accountability pressure has grown, so has the need to define quality in health care services and to develop and implement methods of assessment and assurance. The conceptual dimensions of quality were formulated decades ago (Lee/Jones Report) (3) as: *acceptability, accessibility, availability, compliance, comprehensiveness, coordination, effectiveness, and efficiency.* Such categories can only become useful, however, when operational definitions have been developed which permit objective measurements for each dimension. Even then, since the results of measurement may depend upon the type of evaluation chosen, there may be little correlation between the values arrived at from differing perspectives. Judging the quality of care by measuring consumer satisfaction may produce a very different result than a parallel judgement based on technical evaluation of practitioner performance. The old paradox "the operation was a success but the patient died" illustrates this dilemma of medical care evaluation.

How is Quality Measured?

Quality is measured by evaluation--a judgement of the worth or value of something. Although most adults "evaluate" frequently prior to making a choice (which automobile to purchase, which school to send the children to), such evaluations are often highly subjective. Objective evaluation is regularly displayed in the Consumer Reports magazine, which each month discusses and compares the merits of this or that refrigerator, margarine, or lawnmower. A typical such report lists the evaluation criteria used in the laboratory tests and displays the performance of a number of similar products when tested against these criteria, often indicating a "best buy" automobile tire or toaster oven.

These published reports illustrate basic principles of evaluation: *measures* (benchmarks, standards) must be used, and *measurement* must be performed. Measurement alone only provides a result which raises the question: compared to what? A measure or referent must be used to produce an answer (how tall? how quiet? how cold?). Based upon the referent used, evaluation is commonly divided into *criterion-referenced* and *norm-referenced* systems. In a criterion-referenced system the value obtained by measurement is compared to measures of excellence or optimal values developed by experts and called evaluation "criteria". In a norm-referenced system, the measured value is compared to statistical norms which express mathematically the means and standard errors of referent values. To illustrate the use of referents, let us assume that the legal speed limit of 55 mph is exceeded by most drivers on the freeway, who, in fact, travel at an average speed of 65 mph. A car travelling at 60 mph is exceeding the criterion (55) but is below the norm (65), illustrating the dependence of the evaluation result on the referent used.

In medical care evaluation both types of measures (criteria and norms) are used. Further, medical care evaluation measures are customarily divided into the domains of input, process, and outcome (4). Input standards or criteria (sometimes called structural standards) apply to the resources--manpower, equipment, facilities--available for medical care. Process criteria specify the outputs of medical care--things done to and for the patient--such as radiographs, laboratory tests, days of care in special units, etc. Outcome criteria depict optimal expected health status--the patient care result--at a specified point in time. To illustrate, an input standard might require an electrical defibrillator in the hospital emergency area. A process standard might specify the manner in which the defibrillator is to be used. An outcome standard states the optimal expected effect of defibrillation on the patient.

Each of the three domains of criteria or measures of medical care evaluation possesses limitations:

- Input or structural criteria only prescribe the readiness to perform and therefore represent proxies for actual process and outome. As measures, they can be described as "necessary but not sufficient," having negative value when absent, but limited positive value when present.

• Process criteria are unwieldy evaluation measures because of their complexity and extensiveness, and because "experts" seldom agree on the precise management of clinical problems. Given the empirical nature of medical practice, few scientifically valid process criteria exist. An equal weight of published literature defends each of the several clinical strategies to cope with breast cancer, depression, hypertension, etc. Any set of hypertension criteria comprehensive enough to specify optimal investigation and management might occupy several printed pages and, because of the diversity of the clinical spectrum of hypertension, might be applicable only to a limited number of hypertensive patients.

• Outcome criteria are limited as evaluation measures for medical care because they are inherently insensitive (most people recover no matter which intervention is employed) and because they are dependent on many variables that are extraneous to the process of medical care. If outcome is defined as one's health status at any point in time, such a measure is (in addition to being multidimensional) dependent on many variables, other than the personal health service transaction, which have a profound effect on health status: stress, diet, risky lifestyles, unhealthful personal habits, and inheritance. The health care system is loath to apply evaluation measures that depend on variables beyond its control.

In addition to the limitations of each domain as evaluation measures, there is little similarity in evaluation results using different domains, even in the same group of patients (5). This difference has resulted in a division of rival medical care evaluation factions into "process" and "outcome" camps, producing a spirited rivalry as to which evaluation approach is "correct." McAuliffe's (6) analysis of this rivalry is recommended to serious readers.

The final topic to be discussed in this section is the semantics of medical care evaluation: the distinctions between such terms as *assessment*, *assurance*, and *control*.

• Quality *assessment* is problem-finding, or evaluation. It implies that measures were employed and measurement was used to define and analyze, to *assess* a problem or situation. Assessment does not imply that corrective action has been taken or problems have been solved.

• Quality *assurance* is problem-solving. It implies that action has been taken to guarantee quality, as an extension of an assessment that identified a quality problem.

• Quality *control* is an aggregate of activities (such as design analysis and statistical sampling with inspection for defects) designed to ensure adequate quality in manufactured products (1). Quality control may be difficult to apply to a service, but not impossible.

The most complete of the three concepts is quality *control*, which implies that 1) optimal performance levels have been identified, 2) actual performance levels have been measured and compared to the optimal values, and 3) corrective action has eliminated any discrepancy between optimal and actual levels.

A simple model of a *control* is illustrated by the thermostat, a servo-regulatory mechanism which rests benignly on the inside wall of almost every room or office. The functional components of this control can be seen in Figure 1:

1) A setting knob which permits the operator to specify the optimal or desired value.

2) A measuring device which reports an actual value to the control's "brain."

3. Wires leading to the furnace and to the air conditioning unit, which permit the control to correct any discrepancy between the optimal and actual values.

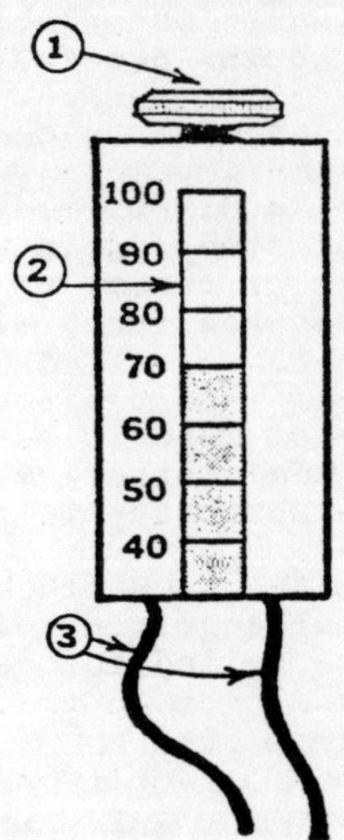

Fig. 1. Functional components of a control

This simple but memorable example services to indicate the components of a quality *control* system for medical care. If we know where we wish to be (setting the knob) and know where we are (measuring actual conditions), we need only an effective action step to control quality of care.

The problems and frustrations of medical care quality control occur in relation to each component and to combinations of components: Recent publications (7, 8) remind us of how few standards we possess which have been validated either by consensus or by scientifically controlled trials. Actual measurement of care quality is frustrated by uneven documentation in record sources and by methodologic problems. Corrective action is blocked by peer protection, fear of legal action, and lack of confidence in the data required to make a judgment. Despite the desire expressed by increasingly informed consumers for quality control in medical care, conceptual and methodologic problems have resulted in the opinion that medical care evaluation and quality assurance activities are ineffective (9).

How is Quality Assured?

The charge of ineffectiveness is based upon the assumption that quality assurance should result in demonstrable evidence of improvement in the quality of patient care. Since this evidence has not been forthcoming except on a sporadic basis, students and proponents of quality assurance feel compelled to attempt to explain the problem. The first hypothesis, that medical care is now perfect, is rejected intuitively. The second hypothesis is that either the problem-finding or the problem-solving steps of the quality control procedure (or both) are faulty.

To be sure, fault can be found with our assessment methods:

1) Medical audit or medical care evaluation has suffered from poor choice of study topic and objectives, poorly drafted or non-discriminating criteria, and the desire of practitioners to paint a rosy picture when faced with the threatening task of self evaluation;

2) review of care in cases of extended hospital stay has been viewed as an administrative, cost-containment problem, rather than as a unique opportunity to identify quality problems;

3) due to the lack of objective methods, reviews of surgical cases, hospital-acquired infections, "incidents," deaths, and other groupings have failed to identify patterns of problems.

Problem-solving (quality *assurance*) activities have been irrelevant or ineffective largely because no problems have been presented to them, or they were disconnected from the problem-finding process.

Substandard medical care might be due to 1) lack of knowledge or skill, or 2) lack of performance. The problem-solving activities designed to correct these two problems are 1) continuing education and 2) credentialing. Unfortunately, both of these quality assurance functions have been less than effective:

1) Continuing education has not been systematically linked up with quality assessment activities, which could provide an agenda of problems in patient care. Lacking such input, continuing medical education (CME) has been directed at perceived needs or has been dedicated to "keeeping up" exercises which are often irrelevant to the (perhaps undiscovered) real needs of practitioners;

2) Credentialing (periodic review of members of the professional staff and assignment of specific clinical privileges to each) has been equally ineffective in assuring quality because it has lacked input from patient care review, which could objectively depict ongoing practitioner performance.

The sentinel problem with quality assurance, then, has been a lack of coordination between problem-finding and problem-solving. The diagram in Figure 2 portrays an integrated system, with the problems identified by quality assessment being directed to the appropriate means of quality assurance.

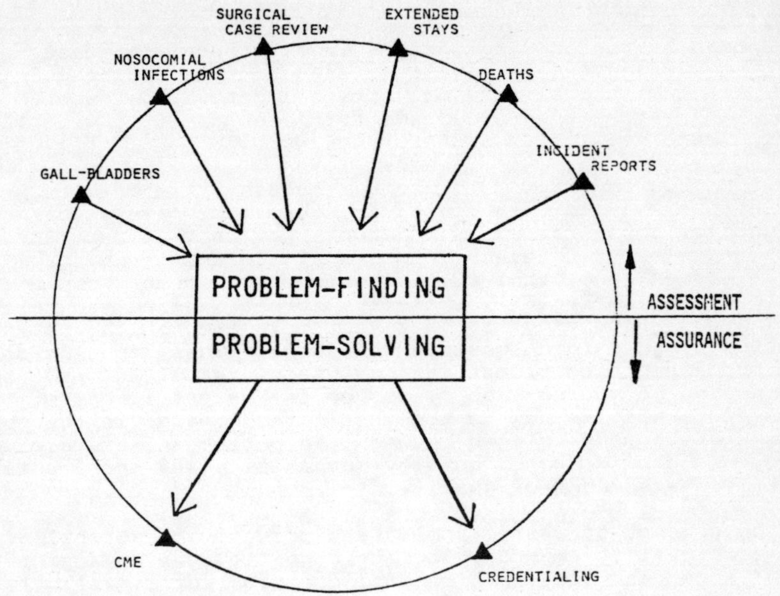

Fig. 2. An integrated quality assurance system

In this "cat's cradle" of activities, assurance of quality depends on 1) a relevant and dynamic program of continuing education responding to lacks in knowledge and skill that have been identified through the review of patient care, and 2) a data-based credentialing process which continually adjusts the clinical privileges of practitioners according to the quality of their performance in patient care. Such a system is suggested by the standards of the JCAH (10) but is rarely accomplished in actual practice.

The Locus of Quality Assurance

Assuming that health care quality can be defined, assessed, and even assured, who should do it? As health care has been increasingly financed from public sources, the accountability of health care providers to the public has increased. Over the years, government has supported the idea of a right to health care by passing laws aimed at providing equal access to health care services of high quality. Governmental support for an ongoing program of basic and applied biomedical research has continued since the creation of the National Institutes of Health in the mid-forties. The Hill-Burton legislation of 1946 provided federal funds for hospital construction and modernization. Government has subsidized the training of health manpower through successive versions of the Health Professions Educational Assistance Act, beginning in 1963. Economic barriers to health care were attacked by providing tax exemptions for employer-sponsored health insurance and, for the poor, unemployed, and aged, by the Medicare and Medicaid legislation of the mid-sixties. Finally, the federal government underwrote its commitment to quality care by passing legislation in 1974 requiring that care conform to professionally developed standards as a prerequisite to reimbursement with public funds. States, meanwhile, enacted legislation which established standards for licensure of a wide variety of health care facilities and professionals.

It is noteworthy that government, through all these legislative interventions, has acted as catalyst, observer, payer, guarantor--a third party role--rather than direct provider. Except for operating hospitals for veterans, members of the uniformed services, merchant seamen, and other special groups, government has avoided the direct provider role. Similarly, it has avoided the role of quality judge, accepting the fact that only the health professions can identify and enforce quality standards. This function of the health professions to promote and maintain ethical and professional standards is, of course, deeply rooted in the traditions of the professions. What is new in the last three decades is the construction of tenuous bridges between the public and private sectors to produce a public accountability mechanism based upon professionally derived standards of quality.

As the concept of shared public and private accountability for health care quality emerged, society began to seek an appropriate locus of accountability. If medical care in Peoria, Illinois is substandard, who should rectify the situation? Several candidates emerge:

- The state licensing authority could theoretically control the quality of care by licensing only those facilities and practitioners who exceed a threshold level of competence or performance. While minimal essential structural criteria could be used in the licensing of facilities, the states have no means of evaluating professional performance on an ongoing basis. Licensure has been based upon a one-time appraisal of an applicant's supply of knowledge by means of a written examination. Licenses have been renewed by certifying attendance at postgraduate education programs and payment of a fee.

- Professional credentialing (certification, registry and the like) holds no more promise than licensing as a means to assure that health professionals exceed certain competence or performance levels. Although the various professional credentialing boards seeks to correct the obvious flaw of assuming lifetime competence on the basis of a single assessment, they cannot avoid the flaw which in the public's view is most serious: that professional certification is voluntary.

- State health departments test and certify water supplies and restaurants but, alas, have no mandate (or data base) to certify professional performance.

- Medical schools are proud of their favorite sons, who have become famous scientists and brilliant technicians, but claim no responsibility for the lowest quartile of graduates who barely exceed(if at all) minimal levels of competence.

• Organizations of health professionals (such as county medical societies) are responsive to public complaints about fees, ethics, and bizarre physician behavior, but like other professional bodies have no data base by which to judge the clinical performance of any of their members. They, too, suffer from the fatal limitation that membership is voluntary.

• Of all the potential candidates to exercise accountability for health care, one stands out--*the hospital*--on the basis of several characteristics: 1) a tradition of public accountability by virtue of its licensed status and community board of trustees; 2) excellent documentation of medical care transactions; 3) a professional staff organization to provide the peer forum necessary for review and evaluation; and 4) administrative support and organizational know-how provided by highly professionalized management. The hospital's own professional staff credentialing process corrects many of the flaws of the process outside the hospital: Unlike licensure, clinical privileges are limited to the area most relevant to competence according to education and previous experience; unlike certification, professional staff credentials are mandatorily reviewed every two years; and unlike both licensure and certification, hospital credentialing is based on periodic reappraisal of practitioner performance.

In addition, the two major mechanisms of public accountability are directed at the hospital: Professional Standards Review, mandated by PL 92-603, utilizes a delegation process which makes the individual hospital the unit of accountability. Likewise, the JCAH focuses on the individual hospital in applying its professionally developed standards designed to maintain and promote the "optimal achievable" quality of patient care.

Alternatives to Professional Involvement

In conclusion, it is important to indicate to health care practitioners why they should be involved in quality assurance activities. Many of them are too busy giving care to devote the time and energy required to evaluate care effectively, which is another way of saying that they are not convinced of the importance of evaluation. However, the current cost crisis and quality crisis make health care evaluation by professionals doubly urgent.

The cost crisis is exemplified by the cost of a day in the hospital, which, for the average acute care "general" hospital, is about $200 per day and rising at the alarming rate of 15% per annum, leading to forecasts of a $1000 per diem by 1988 (11). The per capita cost for health care is around $800 per year, calculated by dividing the total U.S. health care bill of almost $200 billion by the population. The Medicare/Medicaid program cost $1.2 billion in 1966, the first year of implementation. Current projections for Medicare are $34 billion per annum, and Medicaid adds an almost equal amount when both federal and state expenditures are calculated. Health policy analysts consider the rate of cost escalation to be the most serious crisis in the current litany of woes of the health care system.

Simultaneously, there is mounting evidence of a quality crisis in health care. The quality of care provided to inner city recipients of publicly-funded health programs is so low that such programs have been pejoratively described as "Medicaid mills." Lawsuits claiming professional negligence have escalated to the point where professional liability insurance is either prohibitively expensive or unavailable at any cost, a situation referred to as the "malpractice crisis." From a review of 20,000 medical records, a recent California study concluded that "potentially compensable events" occurred with a frequency of 5% in hospitalized patients (12). It is alleged that unnecessary surgery is so rampant that 11,800 U.S. women die annually as a result of unnecessary hysterectomies. These and other data reporting wide variations in surgical procedures have led private and public third parties to instigate "second opinion" programs prior to elective surgery. Finally, there is mounting public concern about and professional response to the problem of the "impaired physician," one who, because of senility, chemical dependency, or behavioral and other mental disorders, is vulnerable to altered professional performance.

The present cost and quality crises should convince us that 1) society cannot tolerate rampant inflation in health prices much longer, 2) limited resources should be distributed according to optimal cost-effectiveness, and 3) public policy decisions about quality, cost/quality tradeoffs and the like require professional input. This last need is frustrated by the reluctance of practitioners to become involved, a reluctance which stems from several factors: 1) practitioners are not taught to be evaluators during their professional training, 2) concepts such as quality assurance, cost-benefit, and performance evaluation are exceedingly complex and are limited by the state of the art, and 3) a practitioner willing to become involved may find himself the subject of a lawsuit by a colleague who feels he was treated unfairly.

Despite this perhaps understandable reluctance on the part of health practitioners, the problems will not go away. If health professionals fail to get involved in quality assessment and assurance, the standards of care and their enforcement will pass to judges and juries for arbitration. If health professionals avoid a role in cost containment and cost benefit matters, decisions about price and resource allocation will be made by third parties.

There is at least a vaguely perceived lull in the malpractice crisis; various actions of state legislatures are creating a climate of immunity by attempting to limit claims, truncate the statute of limitation, etc. These legislative actions are society's response to the threat of disruption in medical care occasioned by the spectre of professional liability. But no group, not even health care professionals, can expect special treatment under the law--the *quid pro quo* for statutory immunity is a vigorous and effective response by professionals to the quality crisis.

In a very real sense, today's health professional is a "double agent," one who is publicly accountable for the quality and cost of publicly financed care, and at the same time the defender of the patient's right not to be harmed by arbitrary or capricious allocation of resources.

Summary

The aim of this paper has been to present the following points:

1) Despite conceptual and methodologic problems, the quality of medical and other health care can be assessed (evaluated).

2) Quality assessment can be transformed into quality assurance or control by appropriate action, even though much of the initial activity in medical quality assurance has been ineffectual and has lacked coordination.

3) Public accountability for the cost and quality of care has increased in proportion to public financing of care.

4) The locus of accountability for both the cost and quality of health care services is and should be the hospital, due to its ability to develop standards, review and evaluate care, and implement remedial action.

5) The significant problems of both cost and quality in health care which will not go away just because health practitioners are reluctant to become involved. Other-than-professional initiatives will fill the void, perhaps to the detriment of patients and the public.

REFERENCES

1. Merriam-Webster, Webster's New Collegiate Dictionary. G. & C. Merriam Company, Springfield, Massachusetts, (1977).

2. Pirsig, Robert M., Zen and the Art of Motorcycle Maintenance. Bantam Books, New York, (1976).

3. Lee, R.I., et al., The Fundamentals of Good Medical Care. University of Chicago Press, Chicago, (1933).

4. Donabedian, A. Evaluating the quality of medical care, Milbank Mem. Fund. Quart. 44:166, (1966).

5. Brook, Robert H., Quality of care assessment: choosing a method for peer review. New Engl. J. Med. 288:1323, (1973).

6. McAuliffe, W.E., Studies of process-outcome correlations in medical care evaluation: a critique. Med. Care 16:907, (1978).

7. Carden, T.S., Tonsillectomy -- trials and tribulations: a report on the NIH consensus conference on indications for T & A. J. Amer. Med. Assn. 240:1961, (1978).

8. Greenberg, Robert A., et al., Physician opinions on the use of antibiotics in respiratory infections. J.A.M.A. 240:650, (1978).

9. Assessing Quality in Health Care: An Evaluation, Institute of Medicine, IPM 76-04, (1976).

10. Accreditation Manual for Hospitals, Joint Commission on Accreditation of Hospitals, Chicago, Illinois, (1980).

11. State of Connecticut, Commission on Hospitals and Health Care, Third Annual Report to the Governor and General Assembly, January 1, (1977).

12. Report on the Medical Insurance Feasibility Study, California Medical Association, (1977).

Discussion of Fifer's "Quality Assurance in Health Care"

William M. Goldberg, M.D.

In his discussion, 'What is Quality? How do we measure it?' Dr. Fifer commented that organizations such as airlines and those producing Coca Cola and Tetracycline assure a degree of quality and adhere to certain standards. These areas all have a defined product. I think the problem facing us in assessing the quality of hospital or doctor's care is that we have not defined our actual product. This makes it difficult to describe the methods that produce quality, and also makes it difficult to set standards.

I feel that the medical product is not so much a lack of disease, but a lack of illness behavior. As we all know, there are very few situations in which we can effect complete cures, coming out with a patient free of any disorder or disease. In the surgical specialities it is a little easier to say, for example, that the end result will be an appendix-free patient without any morbidity or mortality. However, in most clinical situations we have to study illness behavior.

Since illness behavior affects a person's ability to carry on a normal lifestyle, our desired outcome might be a patient able to return to work or to a normal lifestyle. For many years we have been so involved with the disease process that we have forgotten the illness state; we have tried to be curers of disease rather than healers of the sick. We must now concentrate on producing patients with less illness even though we may not be able to cure their diseases.

If we define our product as a lack of illness behavior, and our most desirable outcome a return to work, then the most undesirable result would be total disability. According to statistics recently published in the New York Times (1), annual disability payments in the United States have increased from 500 million dollars in 1960 to 16 billion dollars in 1979; projected spending by the year 1985 is 27 billion dollars. During this same time span, the number of people on insurance disability payments will have also increased from 500,000 to 4 million. At the present time there are approximately 3 million people in the United States who can be considered totally disabled since they are receiving disability insurance. This does not make sense, because during the past twenty years we have improved medical care and thus should have less disease. No new major diseases have developed, yet we end up with more disabled patients, more people on disability insurance, and, therefore, more patients demonstrating illness behavior. One of our goals then, has to be patients demonstrating little illness behavior: off disability insurance, returning to work and to an active, normal lifestyle. Returning home, to the outside world, is not enough. In any hospital assessment method, determining outcome must be built into our quality audit methods.

How do we evaluate outcome, and who should do it? I agree with Dr. Fifer that it cannot be left up to the medical societies or to the government. Evaluation has to be a function of an organization within the individual hospital or the individual community. I personally feel that the quality of care must be determined by organization of peers within each region, involving all hospitals as well as outpatient facilities. The hospital seems to be the easiest place to start, since we are doing all our present medical audits there. However, these reviews only seem to work well when we can audit specific procedures such as surgery, or treatment of defined diseases such as pneumonia and myocardial infarction. I think this approach is worthwhile, but in most instances it does not really consider the total illness state.

How can we possibly improve the situation when we take illness behavior into account? We can do this by decreasing the sick role the patient adopts while in hospital. It seems to me that each hospital should be divided into functional units which would maintain a link with the patient after he leaves hospital. I think the patient must be admitted to hospital for specific reasons and be put into a unit where therapy is carried out in the most efficient fashion, and then be discharged. There must be a follow-up, a linkage of the inpatient part of the treatment with an ongoing outpatient program that results in lessened illness behavior and the final desired outcome of a return to a normal lifestyle and a return to work.

For example, a patient is admitted to a cardiology unit and treated in the appropriate fashion for heart disease. When discharged, on the proper medications, he would know how to take these medications, and there would be a proper follow-up ensuring consistent use with no undesirable side effects. A plan would be carried out to encourage nearly normal activity and, ultimately, the return to work. In many hospitals at present, a Coronary Care Unit patient is treated perfectly well, but is discharged home not knowing what medications to take, and is often not advised when and how to return to work or to begin an exercise program; the patient often ends up with major illness behavior although the organic aspect of the disease was well treated. One could find similar examples in other hospital areas. Thus, if the whole hospital were organized by functional units, each unit would have a mandate to attack the patient's problem and lessen the sick role while in hospital, and to establish a link through an outpatient follow-up program which would encourage loss of illness behavior and resumption of a normal lifestyle, the ultimate goal.

Another important way to ensure the best quality of care in hospital is to make quality control the major responsibility of the chiefs of divisions or heads of services. They should see that work of high quality is carried out in each department in an effective, efficient, and economical fashion, following guidelines laid down by a departmental peer group. In too many teaching institutions, the heads of service or chiefs of divisions have education and research as their major role; in non-teaching institutions these are mainly honorary positions of ill-defined responsibility. In both instances heads and chiefs must be rewarded less for service than for their role in quality control. It seems to me that if this were the main role of these individuals supposedly in charge, their staffs would be less likely to develop poor habits in the practice of medicine, surgery, and other specialities. There was the notorious 'Nork Case' in California, where the court showed that the doctor had carried out an atrocious orthopedic surgical procedure while working in an institution which had the proper appraisal procedures. The tissue committees and other standing committees related to quality of care in no way eliminated the poor care that this individual surgeon delivered. Obviously, in that hospital, the whole process was more theoretical than applied: no one was taking the responsibility either to ensure some quality control of care, or to carry out the principles that had been laid down by the various committees. Unfortunately, at the present time many of our quality assessment and audit committees study process more than the delivery of actual care. In addition, they are more interested in immediate hospital results than long-term outcome.

The other broad areas that should be studied in relation to quality control or quality assessment in our hospitals are the use of drugs and investigational procedures. For example, in our institution, Dr. M. Achong (2) studied a group of elderly patients who were considered to be depressed, and were awaiting placement in extended care facilities. This group of 82 patients had been described as markedly or extremely depressed at the time of referral to our service, and yet 14 received prescriptions for hypnotic sedative agents, 8 received prescriptions for major tranquilizers, and only 1 received a prescription for an antidepressant. It would therefore appear that even in hospitals with good medical audit and quality assessment procedures, markedly depressed patients who should be receiving antidepressants, sometimes do not. An overview of patients in three institutions in Hamilton suggests that doctors think they are using antidepressants logically, but they are not. We intend to inform the medical staffs of these results, and see if the situation improves. Dr. Achong (3, 4) did a similar study on the rational use of prophylactic antibiotics in our institution and found that they were not used appropriately. This report was then circulated to the members of the staff. A reassessment two years later showed a marked improvement in the medical staff's performance. This indicates that if you study broad areas, find specific reversible problems, and then inform the staff and the heads of services, performance can improve. This same process could easily be applied to the use of investigational tools such as radiological procedures and laboratory tests.

Another problem I think we must face in the quality of practice of medicine, surgery, psychiatry, or any of the specialities is the present reward system. We reward doctors more for doing things than for not doing things: running tests, admitting patients to hospital, performing surgery. In no way do we, from a psychological point of view, "punish" doctors for carrying out unnecessary tests or procedures; on the contrary, we reward them financially. It seems to me that somehow we have to reward doctors for good outcomes and for lessened illness behavior in their patients, and somehow punish them for carrying out unnecessary tests and for ineffective procedural therapy.

Similarly, we financially reward patients for being ill and for adopting a sick role. The New York Times article cited earlier (1) pointed out that many patients on disability insurance receive nearly the same amount of money when they are not working as when they were working. In addition, if they were well, many of them would be punished by having to go back to jobs which they found distasteful. Thus, the present system actually rewards people for being disabled. I do not know what other rewards are received by the very miserable and unhappy disabled patients that we see. Somehow, we must have fewer rewards for the sick role, fewer rewards for illness behavior, and more rewards for being well and active and for carrying out normal activities. Somehow we must have a built-in punishment--in a psychological or a financial sense--for demonstrating illness behavior.

In the long run, we will only accomplish our goal of quality of care if our undergraduate and postgraduate training fosters an attitude of self-criticism and an acceptance of peer criticism in our new doctors. We must train students in an atmosphere where quality assessment of their work is essential, and where a healthy, illness-free outcome is their ultimate goal, not just the absence of disease. In medical education, we are continually stressing that our students should have a lifelong attitude towards learning. What is equally important is that they develop a lifelong attitude of self-criticism, welcoming at all times, and in an open fashion, peer review of their work. We must not train them in an environment where their role models, while usually very capable, are often opinionated and closed to criticism; we should expose our students to individuals who demonstrate an attitude of self-criticism and who welcome peer assessment of their own clinical activities.

REFERENCES

1. Cowan, E., New York Times, Sunday, February 25 (1979).

2. Achong, M.R., Bayne, J.R.D., Gerson, L.W., Golshani, S., Prescribing of Psychoactive Drugs for Chronically Ill, Elderly Patients. Can. Med. Assoc. J., 118; 1503-1508 (1978).

3. Achong, M.R., Wood, J., Theal, H.K., Goldberg, R., Thompson,D. A., Changes in Hospital Antibiotic Therapy after a Quality of Use Study. Lancet, 2; 1118-1122, (1977).

4. Achong, M.R., Hauser, B.A., Klusky, J.L., Rational and Irrational Use of Antibiotics in a Canadian Teaching Hospital. Can. Psychiatr. Assoc. J., 116; 256-259, (1977)

Ten Assumptions Which Cripple Psychiatrists' Participation in Quality Assurance Activities

Alex Richman, M.D.*

This paper discusses the drastic changes in self-assessment which have occurred within psychiatric agencies over the years, outlines various aspects of QUALITY ASSURANCE, and presents ten assumptions which cripple the participation of psychiatrists in clinical care evaluation studies.

The Tradition of Self-Assessment and Self-Correction

Scrutiny of the work of psychiatrists is not new. As an integral part of professional practice, psychiatrists traditionally have been responsible for assessing and correcting their own work as well as the work of colleagues. In addition, within clinical agencies, psychiatrists have been responsible for supervising the caseloads of others, maintaining high standards and high quality care, defining clinical policies and procedures, and evaluating the professional qualifications and competence of applicants to the medical staff.

Many years ago, Adolph Meyer (1) emphasized that psychiatrists must show "that the right thing is done when it is needed", that physicians should consider the therapeutic indications, expectations, and actual results of treatment, and should be involved in the active review of treatment of individual patients. In the early 1900's, when requirements for reviewing patient care were implicit, the review was carried out in an informal manner and not documented. What has changed?

The Garden of Eden of Mental Health Services

In the distant past, there was a Garden of Eden for mental health services. Today, there may still be some mental health services which resemble that Garden of Eden.

---

* The assistance of Mrs. B. Brunelle and the National Health Research and Development Program (6603-1115-48) is acknowledged.

The mental health Garden of Eden had outstanding staff, clear organizational structure and goals, and explicit procedures for clinical supervision and systematic review of the professional work. The staff were skilled and satisfied; they remained in the setting in which they had been trained. The expectations for patient care were clear; a practitioner not only understood what was expected of him, but how his colleagues in psychiatry and other disciplines would act.

From year to year, although clinical innovations were adopted and shared by the staff, the treatment philosophy remained internally coherent. Different clinical problems were treated in different ways; rarely would similar problems be treated by apparently different approaches. There were obvious differences between practitioners in emphasis but not in therapeutic philosophy. Who did what to whom, and why, was obvious to all professional staff. In contrast to today, there was consensus among the agency staff and continuity over time in the understanding of clinical problems.

Communication between staff, disciplines, and hierarchical levels was effective. The agency's policies and clinical procedures for care and supervision were well defined. In this Garden of Eden, all staff members felt that they shared in decision making and contributed to clinical successes. These feelings of professional pride and clinical prowess were complemented by a continuing process of self-assessment and self-correction.

In the clinical Garden of Eden, professionals from other disciplines helped develop a clinical formulation and comprehensive treatment plan. There was clear demarcation as to which practitioner was responsible for each patient. Treatment was focused on goals defined in the treatment plan; clinical progress was periodically reviewed and the treatment plan was revised as necessary. The patient and therapist had congruent concerns and treatment expectations. The clinical record, which more than satisfied legal requirements, was occasionally used to jog the practitioner's memory. Since most agencies were small, a few people could supervise the work of the staff, review the case records and be familiar with the clinical status of other practitioners' patients. Clinical and administrative responsibilities were clearly defined. Clinical policies and procedures were maintained and modified through close continuing contact of the staff with one another. Problems in patient care were readily visible, frequently discussed, and corrected rather than perpetuated. All went well.

How is Quality Assurance Professed to Occur Today?

High standards of care and supervision are maintained in an ineffable manner. Everyone feels that problems are rare. The agency runs smoothly--almost as well as the private office of a solo practitioner. Utilization is high; staff are busy; patients generally respond to treatment. Rarely are there complaints from patients or the community. The staff, who come from diverse settings, quickly absorb procedures and policies which have no need to be written down; newcomers, by means of hints, nudges, and informal contacts, learn what is expected. At the same time, the agency, which has no systematic procedure for orienting staff, is too complex to be readily understood by outsiders. The ways in which the clinical staff work together, the division of tasks, the mechanisms for supervision, direction, and decision making are quite informal; because they work so well, there is little need for documentation or formal discussion. There are many potential opportunities to discuss cases, to review old programs, and to solve the sporadic problems which might arise. It is hardly ever necessary to take time from clinical work to hold committee meetings of the staff. Occasional problems in patient care, upon very thorough and impartial review, are found to be the difficulties which often occur in patients with mental disorders, complications which may be expected no matter what the treatment or who the practitioner, unfortunate occurrences which are seen in the best of clinics and hospitals.

Members of the clinical staff are preoccupied with their responsibilities for patient care and the burden of their case load. If their case load were reduced or the demands for therapy lessened, then it would be justified to spend more time in being concerned with the over-all management and organization of their clinical agency, in the in-service training and didactic supervision of new graduates, and in orienting other staff to newer ideologies and therapies which arise among practitioners who have diverse backgrounds, different ideologies, and a pot pourri of approaches to clinical care.

Although many disciplines, therapeutic approaches, and individual interests are represented, each staff member has met the requirements for an academic degree, membership in a professional society, has attended workshops and professional meetings, or has seriously studied the writings of some of the leading therapists in the field today. It is not difficult to determine the qualifications of the staff from their diplomas, professional licenses, bookshelves, or the professional way in which they describe their clinical work.

From time to time, there are case conferences or clinical discussions which substantiate the individual and general awareness that definite diagnosis of a complex case is difficult, and that therapists of equal skill and experience may handle the same case in totally different ways. The subtleties of clinical problems and the sensitivities of clinicians cannot be adequately detailed in the clinical record, which already contains too much personal data for a confidential file.

Despite these difficulties, there is considerable trust and understanding. Because of the close contact with one another, staff are well able to understand how each clinician can individually contribute to clinical excellence and how diversity enhances the eclectic, dynamic approaches of their particular setting.

Systematic review of patient progress is covered within the supervisory chain for new graduates. Each discipline head is well able to monitor the work of his staff and to continuously propound the never-ending need for additional staff. Review of clinical records is largely the responsibility of the medical records staff, and is well known to be a holding-operation until a new approach is developed for content, dictating, transcribing, and retrieving.

Occasionally, researchers or program evaluators try to apply textbook approaches which do not take into account the unique features of the clinic, the difficulties of individualizing treatment, or the long-term perspective required to assess meaningful change. Sporadically, some staff members might attempt to change the system for clinical records, supervision, or committee work, but these efforts are usually short-lived because of their interference with direct clinical care.

In most agencies the clinical staff are able to focus their efforts on their direct clinical work and do not have to divert their attention to questions of quality, self-assessment, or self-correction. These tasks are performed implicitly by those designated as supervisors or discipline heads, who do not want to become preoccupied with the difficulties of reviewing clinical records, the relation of team discussion to patients' response, or the documentation of well understood and uniformly practiced procedures.

During the month before the visit of the Accreditation surveyors, the policy and procedure manuals presented at the time of the last Accreditation survey are resurrected, or are borrowed from other agencies and rapidly duplicated. Although outside surveyors are concerned with many topics during their one or two day visit, practitioners have little chance to communicate their need for more time to maintain high quality work. To the practitioner, the process of systematic assessment is uncongenial--adverse to feelings, to habits, to everyday work; it is an imposed and ungrateful duty, (2). Among the clinical staff, there is little discussion of mistakes or failures.

Bite the Apple, or Bite the Bullet

One day, new requirements unexpectedly appear for reasons previously hidden from the staff--accountability, decreased public trust, third-party payers, legal responsibilities of the Governing Board, loss protection, etc. The red tape hits the fan.

The process notes used for training and supervision are, by themselves, considered insufficient. Each patient must have a clinical record, and these records must be reviewed to see whether they are complete and whether their content justifies the diagnosis and treatment plan. Clinical policies and procedures, although well understood by all, must be documented. The traditional system for case load supervision must be defined and its operation documented.

The requirement which is most difficult for the staff is that they document the process of professional self-assessment and self-correction by means of a clinical care evaluation study. Now, requirements for review are explicit, the procedures are specified, and professionals are required to document the ways in which the review is performed and reported (3).

Quality of Care

QUALITY OF CARE encompasses many topics. It may be measured in terms of technical competence, humanity, need, acceptability, appropriateness, inputs, structure, process, or outcome by using standards, criteria, norms, or direct quantitative or qualitative measures (4).

There is no universal definition of QUALITY. The meaning varies in different contexts, or between discussants in the same context. Without initial agreement of what is meant by QUALITY, further discussion is impossible. Table 1 is a roster of items useful for clarifying in advance which aspect of QUALITY is being discussed (5).

My discussion of QUALITY ASSURANCE does not encompass all aspects of QUALITY, but is focussed on the Clinical Care Evaluation Study of the PSRO, JCAH, or CCHA type. This specific approach can be documented (#20), involves screening criteria (#49), is reported to the Governing Board (#47), can measure change (#29), is performed by the organized professional staff (#33), includes peer review (#37b), is one of the methods for professional self-scrutiny/self-correction (#51), is an audit of the agency's organization and compliance with written policies and procedures (#4b), but is NOT a panacea (#35) to satisfy multiple requirements for staff supervision, setting and maintainence of standards, concurrent (utilization) review, reviewing the completeness of clinical records, etc., etc.

What Is Quality Assurance?

QUALITY ASSURANCE is more than peer review. Review occurs at various levels: between colleagues, within case load supervision, by service chiefs and staff committees. Peers apply professional experience and judgement to formally assess the "worth" or "QUALITY" of another professional's work. Rarely are these forms of peer review explicit, subject to documentation, or focussed on a defined topic. Usually, the "QUALITY" of work is assessed subjectively, unsystematically, and in global terms. In order to make peer review more effective, it is necessary to have structure, focus, and protection for the reviewers.

Even when peer review is focussed within committees concerned with specific topics such as complaints from patients and untoward occurrences, review is usually unsystematic and rarely results in identification and elimination of substandard performance (6). Follow-up of recommendations is unusual. The framework of clinical care evaluation studies provides structure, focus, and protection, as well as efficiency and effectiveness.

The clinical care evaluation study is confused with other types of review activities. There are many kinds of systematized review activities which differ in what is being reviewed, who is doing the review, and the basis of the review (7). Figure 1(p.25) illustrates some of the review activities with which clinical care evaluation studies are confused.

TABLE 1

A list of inter-related but diverse topics
A roster for focussing discussion on "Quality" -
A tower of Babel

1. Accountability
2. Accreditation
3. All/Some (Sample)
4. Audit -
   a) Clinical Records Completeness
   b) Agency's organization and compliance to policies and procedures
5. Claims Review
6. Clinical Care Evaluation -
   a) Case Conferences
   b) Treatment Committees
   c) Case load Supervision
   d) Clinical Care Evaluation or Study(PSRO;JCAH;AC/PF;CCHA types)
   e) Clinician's close scrutiny of records
   f) Research
7. Clinical Guidelines (Algorithm)
8. Clinical Judgement
9. Clinical Trial, Randomized
10. Competency
11. Concurrent Review
12. Confidentiality
13. Consumer Satisfaction
14. Content/Configuration (Process)
15. Continuing Education
16. Cost Containment
17. Credentialling
18. Data Base, Electronic
19. Diagnostic Validity (Diagnostic Criteria)
20. Documentation -
   a) Clinical Record
   b) Case load Supervision
   c) Clinical Care Evaluation Study
21. End result/impact (Outcome)
22. Explicit / Implicit / Criteria
23. Fault Finding/Fixing-(Action Research, Operations Research)
24. Follow-up -
   a) Outcome of Care
   b) Results of Recommendations
25. Governance
26. Level of Care
27. Licensing
28. Management/Information System
29. Measurement
30. Medical/Clinical Model
31. Medical Need
32. Norms
33. Organized Professional Staff
34. Outcome/Process/Structure
35. Panacea--Single Procedure which is Less Work, But Satisfies All External Requirements
36. Patients/Person; Individual/ Aggregate
37. Peer -
   a) Peer Judgement (Review by peers)
   b) Peer Review (systematic, focussed, documented, measurable)
38. Performance Measures
39. Policy Review
40. Problem Solving
41. Procedure Manual
42. Professionalism
43. Profile of Practice
44. Program Evaluation
45. Quality Assurance -
   a) Concept
   b) Objective
   c) Procedures
46. Record Keeping (POMR, etc.)
47. Report to Governing Board
48. Review Activities
49. Screening Criteria
50. Second opinion or consultation
51. Self-scrutiny/Correction
52. Silence - the invisible non-process
53. Standards -
   a) Minimum Standards
   b) Optimal Standards
54. Supervision
55. Text Book
56. Therapy
57. Topic (for patient care evaluation study) -
   a) Diagnosis
   b) Problem in Care
   c) Procedure
58. Threat to Autonomy
59. Treatment Planning
60. Trust
61. Utilization Review (retrospective)
62. Value Judgement
63. Variation -
   etc.
   etc.

DANGER: DO NOT BEGIN DISCUSSION OF "QUALITY" WITHOUT AGREEING IN ADVANCE WHICH OF THE ABOVE ITEMS ARE BEING CONSIDERED !!

CLINICAL RECORD					DATA ABSTRACTS			
SINGLE RECORD		MANY RECORDS		WHAT IS REVIEWED	UNIFORM FORMAT		SPECIFIC FORMAT IN EACH FACILITY	
PRACTITIONER	NON-PRACTITIONERS INITIALLY		PRACTITIONER	WHO REVIEWS	CLERK; TECHNICIAN; PROFESSIONAL	PROFESSIONAL/TECHNICAL STAFF		
IMPLICIT CLINICAL JUDGEMENT	EXPLICIT SCREENING CRITERIA PLUS FOCUSSED PEER REVIEW OF PATIENT RECORDS		CHECK LIST PLUS IMPLICIT CLINICAL JUDGEMENT	BASIS OF REVIEW	CHECK LIST; SCREENING CRITERIA, PEER REVIEW	HIGH LEVELS OF TECHNICAL SKILLS, EXTENSIVE DATA PROCESSING, AND CONSIDERABLE STATISTICAL SOPHISTICATION		
COLLEGIAL RELATIONS	CONCURRENT (UTILIZATION) REVIEW (PSRO TYPE)	CLINICAL CARE EVALUATION (PSRO TYPE)	RECORDS REVIEW	TYPE	CLAIMS REVIEW	PROFILE ANALYSIS (PSRO TYPE)	PROGRAM EVALUATION	MANAGEMENT INFORMATION

Fig. 1, Differences between review activities

QUALITY ASSURANCE is required by accrediting agencies (CCHA,JCAH, ACPF) and state regulations, third party payers and local PSRO's. QUALITY ASSURANCE is a principle, a goal, and a process (8).

The principle is that practitioners are willing to document the extent to which substandard performance is identified and eliminated.

The goal is to find what's wrong and fix it. QUALITY ASSURANCE is a pathway, not a destination; the activity is open-ended. More important than the specific topic is the identification of changes which should be made by staff, administration, or committees of the organized professional staff.

There are many processes for self-assessment and self-correction. The Clinical Care Evaluation Study (patient care evaluation study, medical audit, PSRO retrospective review) is the chief method which can be documented and is measurable. There are other methods concerned with enhancing or assuring "QUALITY" which are not readily documented, are less amenable to measurement, and should not be called QUALITY ASSURANCE.

Psychiatry's Responses to the New Requirements

How has psychiatry responded to the requirements for documenting professional self-assessment and self-correction? With difficulty, reluctance, and misunderstanding; psychiatrists have claimed that the Clinical Care Evaluation Study diminishes the autonomy of the profession, violates confidentiality, reduces time for clinical care, is an "overkill" reaction to a very few "bad apples", is inappropriate for mental disorders, or is an ivory-tower approach which ignores the realities of clinical practice.

As yet, it is still rare for Clinical Care Evaluation Studies to be used 1) to inform staff, and the Governing Board of the agency, about the need for changes by clinicians, administration, or committees of the organized professional staff, 2) to determine whether the organized structure of the hospital or clinic is assigning responsibility and assuming direction to its activities, and 3) to determine whether the informal or formal mechanisms for supervision and self-improvement are working.

There are few published examples of psychiatric Clinical Care Evaluation Studies which conform to the 1979 requirements. Even in regions where there is much external pressure to produce Clinical Care Evaluation Studies, psychiatry lags far behind the other medical specialities which also deal with complex aspects of human behavior.

Basic Assumptions - (none of which are valid)

In psychotherapy, as in science, there are many factors which contribute to conscious and unconscious resistance to change. Psychiatrists refer to these factors as defenses; sociologists refer to them as governing images: summary characterizations organized around a coherent perspective which largely predetermine an individual's behavior (9). This section deals with some of the assumptions held to some degree by many psychiatrists. These assumptions are rarely articulated. They are brought out into the open here to help us understand why QUALITY ASSURANCE procedures have been difficult to apply to psychiatry.

ASSUMPTION 1) "Many roads lead to Rome"

There are many different approaches--ranging from informal chats and corridor consultations to formal case conferences, supervision of videotaped sessions, etc.--any of which will assure QUALITY care.

Psychiatrists are constrained by the lock-step sequence of the Clinical Care Evaluation Study. Since practitioners vary considerably and since the same goal may be attained by quite different approaches, any form of review is bound to improve quality, even if there is no documentation, measurement, report to external groups, or follow-up.

ASSUMPTION 2) A few"bad apples"are the focus of QUALITY assurance

Psychiatric "bad apples" are concentrated in Medicaid mills in metropolitan areas of the United States, and in small, new, understaffed community mental health centers in rural areas of the United States. They can be found among practitioners who have not kept up with the times, or among those who neglect the past and pursue the newest fads.

It is generally felt that nearly all psychiatrists provide consistently high standards of care at all times, for most patients, and under all circumstances.

ASSUMPTION 3) Psychiatrists' care is highly individualized

Clinical management of a single case is affected by myriad factors. It is far too soon to lay down clinical guidelines for the generic management of some of the common clinical problems. Standardized treatment programs are superficial, reducing the physician's therapeutic armamentarium, inhibiting the delicate admixture of experience and sensitivity, reducing the therapist to a mechanic, and denying our basic understanding of the nature of man. Quality care acknowledges individual differences as more important than similarities.

Profiles of psychiatrists' patterns of practice do not reflect the dynamics of patient/therapist fit, ignore the "personal equation", and are heedless of the intricacies of clinical judgement.

ASSUMPTION 4) Self-assessment and self-correction are so ingrained in the everyday work of the inter-disciplinary clinical team that additional QUALITY ASSURANCE procedures are redundant

"The use of the perspectives and ideas of several therapists of varying disciplines on the diagnosis, prescription for treatment, and the therapeutic treatment itself insures against the errors or lapses that unsupervised practitioners may make. Use of the multiple perspective ... establishes an expectation that the results of proposed interventions will be examined subsequently."(10)

ASSUMPTION 5) "Fine fellows do fine therapy"

Training plus specialist's qualifications plus positive personality ensure work of high QUALITY. In one study, psychiatrists felt that people with whom they might enjoy social contact must be the good psychiatrists.

> Psychiatrists cannot observe colleagues working in their offices nor does the theory define definitive even though indirect signs of good therapeutic practice: specific results cannot be clearly connected to the use of specific techniques. Therefore, psychiatrists may have to evaluate each other from what they can observe--actions of colleagues taken in the ordinary course of life. These easily observable personality characteristics become the major criteria used to evaluate colleagues (11).

ASSUMPTION 6) Patient care within a hospital or clinic is, by and large, a variant of private practice by a solo practitioner

The greater the opportunities for one-to-one care in a clinical agency, the higher the QUALITY of care.

> Most psychiatric hospital treatment in this country has been based on the theories and techniques of the office practice of individual psychotherapy. As a result, if a patient requires hospitalization he is apt to automatically get "more of the same" type of therapy he received on the outside (12).

ASSUMPTION 7) The more psychiatric care received, the better the chances for mental health

> Not for the good that it will do
> But that nothing may be left undone
> On the margin of the impossible.
>
> T. S. Eliot, The Family Reunion

It is generally assumed that patients will respond to treatment in time if there are ample opportunities for varying the treatment approaches. Previous responses to earlier treatment should not be used to exclude patients from further treatment. Since it is rarely possible to predict when a patient might respond, practitioners should persist in their therapeutic efforts (13). Attempts to judge whether treatment should be reduced in frequency, intensity, or duration are clinically inappropriate. Patients who have attained a therapeutic plateau, who do not show continuing improvement with additional treatment, are deemed to need more or different treatment.

ASSUMPTION 8) QUALITY ASSURANCE is a "remedy too strong for the disease"

It has long been recognized that "Faith and knowledge lean largely upon each other in the practice of medicine" (14). The clinician often feels a need for certainty--not about every detail of each case but about his total effectiveness; moreover, he needs a sense of sureness about day-to-day decisions (15). Personal experience is the most immediate source of knowledge which a person has; what can a person trust if he can't trust his own experience?(16) The very enthusiasm and confidence of those who conduct any therapeutic regimen have repeatedly been shown to contribute to its success, but this apparently continues to hold true only as long as the confidence is based upon reality (17).

ASSUMPTION 9) A diagnosis of mental disorder in itself justifies treatment and continuing care

A diagnosis of a mental disorder is prescriptive, indicating the need for clinical intervention. There is a call to psychiatrists to develop and offer preventive and therapeutic measures for all the conditions included in DSM-III. Most persons referred to a mental health agency have a diagnosis of mental disorder, are in need of psychiatric care, and psychiatric treatment is justified.

ASSUMPTION 10) There is a double standard

The tendency of physicians to attribute ineffective treatment to others leads to a strong conviction about the efficacy of one's own treatment (18). Measures of "process" are sufficient to assess the QUALITY of one's own work; measures of "outcome" are needed to demonstrate the QUALITY of the work of others (or the worth of QUALITY ASSURANCE).

Proponents of QUALITY ASSURANCE must demonstrate that their procedures are effective and efficient, while practitioners can support their claims of high quality without demonstrating either effectiveness or efficiency.

Conclusion

One hundred and fifty years ago, Nicoll (2) discussed the reports of Medical Commissioners' visits to asylums for the insane in this manner:

> A commissioner would somewhat resemble the surveyor of the highways and turnpikes of some portion of a county, where... on any inspection, he found a few ruts filled up, he would report, "An improving road"; where no accident of breaking down had happened for a twelve-month, "A good road"; and where a post-chaise could get on seven miles an hour, no doubt he would exclaim, with exultation, "An excellent road this!"

Most of the assumptions I have outlined above go back to Nicoll's time. In order to progress further in the care of mental illness as well as in quality assurance, psychiatrists must identify to what extent these assumptions determine their care of patients and their professional behavior. The less influence these assumptions have the greater the chances that psychiatrists can show "that the right thing is done when it is needed".

REFERENCES

1. Meyer, A., Twenty-first Annual Report of the State Commission in Lunacy, Sept. 30, 1909, in The Collected Papers of Adolf Meyer, Vol. II, Johns Hopkins Press, Baltimore, (1951).

2. Nicoll, S.W., Enquiry into the present state of visitation, in asylums for the reception of insane, and into the modes by which such visitation may be improved, 1828 in R. Hunter and I. Macalpine (eds.), Three hundred Years of Psychiatry, 1535-1860, Oxford University Press, (1963).

3. Riedel, D.C., Tischler, G.L., Myers, J. K. (eds.), Patient Care Evaluation in Mental Health Programs, Cambridge, Mass: Ballinger Publishing Co., (1974).

4. Discursive Dictionary of Health Care, Washington: USGPO,(1976).

5. Richman, A., Philosophy, Goals and Concepts of Quality Assurance in Mental Health Services, presented at the Workshop on Quality Assurance, Texas Department of Mental Health and Mental Retardation, Austin, Texas, January 3, (1979).

6. Jacobs, C.M., Christoffel, T. H., Dixon, N., Measuring the Quality of Patient Care: the rationale for outcome audit: Cambridge, Mass: Ballinger, (1976).

7. Richman, A., The differences between Quality Assurance, Records Committee Review, Program Evaluation and Clinical Supervision, etc., Chapter 2 in Quality Assurance in the Ambulatory Setting: Nine Papers (R. S. Kessler, ed.), St. Albans, Vermont State Institutional Industries Press, (1978).

8. Sanazaro, P. J., Quality assurance in ambulatory care: an overview. Chapter 2 in Ambulatory Medical Care Quality Assurance 1977 (Giebink, E. A., White, N.H. (eds.), LaJolla, Calif: La Jolla Health Science Publications, (1977).

9. Room, R., Governing images and the prevention of alcohol problems, Preventive Medicine, 3: 11-23, (1974).

10. Menninger, R. W., What is Quality Care? A clinician's view. Am. J. Orthopsychiat, 47, 476-483, (1977).

11. Kahn-Hut, R., Psychiatric Theory as Professional Ideology, Ph.D. Dissertation, Brandeis University, (1974).

12. Tucker, G. J. and Maxmen, J.S., The practice of hospital psychiatry: a formulation. Am. J. Psychiatry, 130: 887-891, (1973).

13. Richman, A., Cost/benefit analyses of alcoholism and drug abuse treatment programs: The relevance of recidivism and resource absorption, presented at the Annual Meeting American Association for the Advancement of Science, Washington, D.C., (1978).

14. Lantham,P. M., in Familiar Quotations (J. Bartlett, ed., revised by E. M. Beck) 14th edition, Little, Brown and Company, (1968).

15. Group for the Advancement of Psychiatry. Psychotherapy and the Dual Research Tradition. GAP Report No. 73. October (1969)

16. Thorne, F. C., Clinical Judgement, Brandon, Vermont: Clinical Psychology, (1961).

17. Carstairs, G. M., Revolutions and the rights of man. Am. J. Psychiatry, 134: 979-983, (1977).

18. Shapiro, A. K. and Streuning, E. L., A comparison of the attitudes of a sample of physicians about the effectiveness of their treatment and the treatment of other physicians. J. Psychiat. Res. 10: 217-229, (1974).

Discussion of Richman's "Ten Assumptions Which Cripple Psychiatrists' Participation in Quality Assurance Activities"

Michael G. G. Thompson, M.D.

Dr. Richman is to be complimented on his discussion of the assumptions so often made by clinicians when they are forced to consider patient care review systems. To merely add to his list would be a futile exercise. Instead it behooves us to candidly examine the extent to which we have based our own delivery of services on assumptions rather than hypotheses. The experience of one small agency, the West End Creche Child and Family Clinic in Toronto, will serve as an example of a clinic that for both external and internal reasons was forced to examine the assumptions on which its service delivery system and its treatment programs were based. This paper develops a model which can be illustrated using a Venn diagram. It allows the reader to view Dr. Richman's assumptions in the context of an organization's total functioning. The word "assumption" implies a belief based on lack of data, knowledge, or understanding. The person or group using an assumption usually will discourage any questioning of its validity. Though the words assumption and hypothesis both indicate that the statement being made is not proven to be factual, it is only in the latter case, with "hypothesis", that testing the validity of a pronouncement is encouraged. In large mental health centres, as Dr. Richman has emphasized, we tend to make assumptions which seemingly negate the necessity of objective review.

It was this recognition by key members of the board of the West End Creche which led to a re-examination of the clinic's management and clinical systems. In order to do this it was necessary 1) to set down a few basic objectives that would assist management in assessing the functioning of the clinic from a fresh point of view, 2) to clearly identify which assumptions were being made, and 3) to change a selected number of these assumptions to hypotheses in order to test their validity.

At this juncture, the following statement seemed almost self-evident: The objective of any mental health organization, large or small, must be to put the maximum number of available dollars into productive use. The corollary of this proposition is that every inefficient activity uses up limited dollars that otherwise could have been put into productive use in patient care. Thus, it was evident that every aspect of our organization could and should be made to meet the same general set of criteria: that the activity being carried out be effective, efficient with respect to time and cost, and ethical. Also, the methods used to audit any aspect of the patient care delivery system should also meet the criteria; they would have to be in themselves effective, efficient, and ethical.

In the preceding paragraph, the word "organization" has been used rather loosely, on the premise that it doesn't matter where a dollar is wasted--it is always a dollar removed from patient care. It is therefore important to weed out ineffective and inefficient operations, whether they be in administration, feedback and evaluation mechanisms, or direct patient care.

To be efficient and effective in evaluation, it is necessary to have a model of the organization which allows one both to identify past "assumptions" and to set clear objectives for each area of functioning. The model needs to be broad enough to remain valid no matter what is altered in the organization. If this last criterion is not met, the model would not be capable of suggesting equally well all types of additions, deletions, and modifications that an organization might require over time.

The model need only comprise a limited number of areas into which all functions of the organization can be grouped. A simple paradigm to cover all aspects of any mental health organization is contained in the reporter's classic question, "*Who* does *what* to *whom*?" To this we may add, "At what *cost* and with what *effect* in what period of *time*?"

The *who*, *what*, and *whom* of the first part of this question represent staff, methods of accomplishing functions, and patients. The Venn diagram form (Fig. 1) allows us to visualize the relationships between the subgroupings of each of these three areas. That is, each of the subsections: *staff - methods*, *staff - patients*, *patients - methods* and *staff - patients - methods*, can represent one or more functional operations carried out by the mental health organization. Each of these operations can be tested for efficiency and effectiveness. For example, the *staff* (who) section can represent the systems for hiring personnel, performance counselling, staff supervision, and so on. Similarly the *methods* (what) section can represent (administratively) a system for data collection, recording, transcription, and filing. Clinically, it can represent different treatment regimens for a defined diagnostic entity. The *patient* (whom) section can represent the clinic's system for educating the public and potential referral sources concerning the appropriateness of that clinic's services for a specific clientele.

The *who - what* section can represent systems that delineate which types of staff can effectively and efficiently administer which technique (treatment, bookkeeping, etc.). One system fitting this designation would be the system whereby the composition of treatment teams was decided upon. The *who - whom* section would cover systems

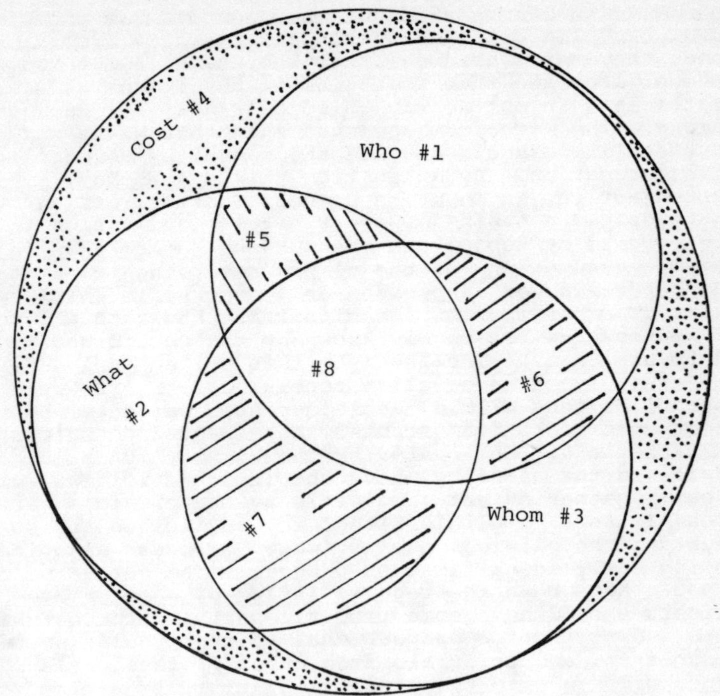

Fig. 1. The Auditing Venn

which monitor the number of hours staff spend in direct patient care as opposed to indirect care (report writing, letter writing, contacts with other agencies, research, education). The *what - whom* section encompasses available and appropriate methods for treating clients, and answers such questions as: "which methods of treatment are best for which groups of clients?" The *who - what - whom* section lies appropriately at the center of the Venn diagram. It represents the most complex systems which include all aspects of patient care. To test the case management system, one must raise such questions as: "Is the balance of expertise on the treatment team sufficient to deliver all the types of treatment necessary for all of the disorders that are referred to the clinic?"

The Venn diagram is very useful for describing an organization in a functional manner: it encourages staff to think in broad all-encompassing terms, while at the same time consciously recognizing previous assumptions in every aspect of their work, and changing these into testable hypotheses. It is, in the final analysis, a method for generating questions which then become hypotheses to test the organization's systems for handling tasks. Two examples may clarify this process.

Example 1: The *whom* section of the Venn diagram prompted the director of our clinic to ask where patients came from. When questioned, the staff "assumed" that they came from throughout the catchment area and that most general physicians and certainly all pediatricians in our nearby children's hospital knew about our services. The director suggested that this might not be so, and that the clinic should examine the system by which clients came to its attention. By definition this system had, like any other, an objective, an input, a process, output, and an evaluation and feedback mechanism. Unfortunately, evaluation and feedback were covered by subjective assumptions rather than objective testing. The assumptions of the clinic regarding its system for obtaining referrals were expressed as a hypothesis which could be tested: "The services of the clinic are known to all potential referral sources and reasonably known by the public who might be expected to use them." The *input* to this system included: the catchment area, location of all potential referral sources, and the number of persons within each diagnostic category who might, from recent epidemiological studies, be expected to suffer from a disorder that could be treated by the clinic. Under *process* were considered the means by which the input activities were carried out: gathering data, advertising the clinic's services (brochures, letters to clinic directors, physicians and so on), and evaluating the clinic's public image. Process also included any existing early identification program. The *output* of this system should have been the regular influx of appropriate clients. These clients should have come from all parts of the catchment areas with a distribution proportional to the population density of each sub-area, and referrals from other professionals should have been appropriate to the population served by each of them. The criteria used for evaluating the effectiveness of this system were the number of referrals from each resource, and the distribution of the client population relative to the general population.

At our clinic when these criteria were applied, it was found 1) that our client population was unevenly distributed relative to the general population, and 2) that even in our largest referral source, a major children's hospital, the large majority of the staff didn't know of us at all, thought we had closed our intake, or thought that we served a different population than we do. These startling facts resulted in a new drive to inform physicians and social workers of our services. Within a few months there was both an increase in appropriate referrals and a more even distribution of clients with respect to the distribution of the population as a whole.

Example 2: In the *who - what - whom* section we asked such questions as: 1) Is the expertise in the clinic balanced and varied enough to offer our clientele all of the most up-to-date methods of treatment? 2) For any selected patient, has a correct diagnosis been made and is an appropriate treatment program being carried out? 3) For the patient population as a whole, have the appropriate steps been taken to arrive at correct diagnoses and treatment plans? 4) For each patient and for their program as a whole, have the staff set goals, criteria to determine whether the goals have been reached, target dates, and methods for attaining the goals? With respect to cost (a circle labelled cost surrounds the entire Venn diagram), the following questions arise: 1) If one changes the composition of the treatment team and therefore alters the methods being used, how will these affect the treatment outcomes of the patients in terms of effectiveness, time efficiency, and cost efficiency? 2) What are the relative costs of treatments on different populations of patients?

Further questions will, of course, arise under the *who - whom - what* rubric, but the questions mentioned above were felt to be most relevant to our clinic, and were given high priority. Since for the most part only assumptions concerning these aspects of care had been made in the past, a new system for investigating each had to be devised and implemented. The clinic turned to the literature and found appropriate methodologies in the "In-depth Patient Care Audit" (1) and the audit system recommended by the Joint Commission on Accreditation of Hospitals (U.S.A.) for evaluating the outcome of clinical care on a large scale (2). When these systems were tested, there were immediate beneficial results. The units were redesigned, and the composition of teams was changed according to new job specifications. The in-depth patient care review audit revealed ineffective multidisciplinary written communication and redundancy in the charting of patients. To remedy this, we introduced a single, comprehensive multidisciplinary conference note, goal attainment scaling, and a new case review system. Even in the initial stages, the setting of team goals resulted in more time spent by the staff in direct patient care and more clients receiving treatment from the clinic.

Further examples could be given for each of the sections of the Venn. However, the important points to emphasize here are: 1) For each area in the Venn diagram, our clinic has asked a number of questions concerning the purposes and effectiveness of procedures being carried out in that area; 2) the Venn diagram as a whole is contained within a circle labelled *cost*, signifying that for every section in it, questions of cost-effective functioning must be raised; 3) each question, whether of procedure or cost, can be expressed as a hypothesis and tested objectively. As many such hypotheses can be generated using the Venn diagram, management and staff must set priorities; only testing which will be cost effective to the organization should be carried out.

From the perspective of this model, Dr. Richman's assumptions seem to be somewhat randomly selected, commonly held assumptions about the functioning of various aspects of the mental health delivery system. These assumptions and many more like them fit logically into the sections of the Venn diagram. For example, assumption #1, "Many roads lead to Rome", includes informal chats, corridor consultations, clinical case conferences, and supervision, and implies that *any* of these ensure quality of care. The corollary for such an assumption could be stated: "A formal clinical audit will not bring about any change in patient care in general nor in the care of randomly selected patients in particular." This is now worded as a testable hypothesis, and fits into the *who - what - whom* section of the Venn. Dr. Richman's assumptions #2 ("A few bad apples are the focus of quality assurance . . ."), #5 ("Fine fellows do fine therapy"), and #8 ("Quality assurance is a remedy too strong for the disease") all fit the general statement "You won't find enough deficiencies in the work at *our* clinic to warrant a clinical audit." This can be translated into a hypothesis: "Examination of patients and their clinical records will show that 100% of essential items and a reasonable percentage of important but not essential items on a comprehensive, clinical audit questionnaire will be fulfilled." This is not supported in practice (1).

Dr. Richman's assumption #3 ("Psychiatric care is highly individualized") is another way of saying that it is not possible to lay down specific guidelines for the general management of problems, and implies that therefore it is not possible to make a list of who is expected to be able to do what and to verify this in some manner in a clinical review. This assumption could be considered in the *who - what - whom* section.

Dr. Richman's assumption #6 implies that one-to-one care represents highest quality treatment. This fits the *what* section and can be altered into a hypothesis: "Individual treatment will have more positive outcomes than other types of care." When stated this way it is a straightforward, much-tested hypothesis with many references in the literature to disprove it.

Dr. Richman's assumption #7 suggests that the more time in treatment, the better the outcome. This fits the *what - whom* section and could be tested by a study of the frequency, intensity, and duration of treatment with respect to treatment outcome.

Dr. Richman's assumption #9 ("A diagnosis of mental disorder in itself justifies treatment and continuing care") fits the *whom* section of the Venn in that it does not require a specific type of professional or specific treatment in order to test it. A corresponding hypothesis might be: "Patients of different diagnostic subtypes who were recommended for an eclectic treatment program within the clinic would have sufficiently positive outcomes to justify the cost and time involved." Interestingly, this was studied at our clinic (3), and the results did not support the assumption.

It becomes clear in examining even such a lengthy list of assumptions as Dr. Richman's that if they are slotted into a framework that encompasses all aspects of the organization, such as the Venn diagram model presented here, entire areas of concern have been omitted, and the assumptions mentioned cover only a small part of the areas into which they fall.

Assumptions appear to be an integral part of everyday clinical functioning. Our experience with them has been threefold. First, discovering what we are covertly assuming is made easier by using a Venn diagram model of the functional structure of the organization; one is forced to think of every system within the organization from a fresh point of view. Second, once some of the assumptions which underlie our administrative and clinical work have been discovered, they can be converted to testable hypotheses. Third, when these hypotheses are tested they are usually found to be at least partly false, and significant changes in the organization and its output ensue.

REFERENCES

1. Thompson, M.G.G., The Clinical Audit in a Psychiatric Setting, Can. Psychiatr. Assoc. J., 22, 261-268, (1977).

2. Joint Commission on Accreditation of Hospitals, Performance Evaluation Procedures for Auditing and Improving Patient Care, Chicago, Illinois, (1971).

3. Havelkova, M., Follow-up Study of 71 Children Diagnosed as Psychotic in Preschool Age, Am. J. Orthopsychiat., 38: 846-851, (1968).

Evaluation of Patient Care and Hospital Accreditation

Henry B. Durost, M.D.

While this paper is being written from the perspective of the Canadian Council on Hospital Accreditation, it is only proper to acknowledge a North American background for the development of the hospital accreditation process. Based on concepts developed by committees of the Clinical Congress of Surgeons of North America, the Hospital Standardization Program was established by the American College of Surgeons in 1918. Members of the nursing discipline should be gratified by the fact that more than half a century earlier, Florence Nightingale had conducted studies of the quality of care available to the British Army during the Crimean War (1).

In 1951 the Joint Commission on Accreditation of Hospitals (J.C.A.H.) was created, the founding sponsors being the American College of Surgeons, the American College of Physicians, the American Hospital Association, the American Medical Association, and the Canadian Medical Association. The latter represented the component organizations of the Canadian Commission on Hospital Accreditation, viz. the Canadian Medical Association, the Royal College of Physicians and Surgeons of Canada, l'Association des Médecins de Langue Française du Canada, and the Canadian Hospital Association. The Canadian Nurses' Association joined the Council in the early 1970's.

By 1958 only 37% of Canadian hospitals had acquired accreditation status. The Joint Commission published no literature in French, and perhaps because the Canadian members of the Joint Commission may have been suffering from the national malady of identity diffusion, the Canadian Council on Hospital Accreditation separated from the Joint Commission and assumed full responsibility for accrediting Canadian hospitals in January 1959.

The Joint Commission and the Canadian Council have worked closely together since the latter assumed an independent status. Standards and procedures have varied slightly, but essentially remained the same. In 1971 the Joint Commission implemented a new set of standards based on optimal, rather than minimal concepts, and in its 1972 Guide to Accreditation of Hospitals the C.C.H.A. followed suit.

Both the C.C.H.A. and J.C.A.H. originally focused on structural variables and credentials as indices of the quality of care being provided, based on the assumption that "if you had good people working in a good environment, together with a good organization, you would produce good care" (2). They have since recognized the limitations of this approach. This paper will discuss the steps taken by the hospital accrediting bodies to develop better standards and to apply them to health care evaluation.

Standards

Tissue committees were originally established to evaluate process aspects of the quality of patient care, but they did not deal with the problem of assessing medical and surgical cases which did not yield tissues, and had little to offer to the assessment of psychiatric care. Review of clinical records by medical audit committees was encouraged, but contained many inherent defects: subjective (implicit) standards, uncontrolled personality variables, and a lack of prior agreement on objective (explicit) standards.

Deficiencies of the chart review system of audit as well as concurrent developments in the field of quality assessment of patient care led the C.C.H.A. to establish new standards, which were published in the 1977 Guide to Hospital Accreditation (3). Standard V states: "The medical staff shall ensure the quality of professional care provided to patients in the hospital by continual review and evaluation of the overall patterns of clinical practice, of the clinical activities of individual members, and of the ultimate effectiveness of the patient care rendered."

Interpretation of this Standard includes the following statements:

"Professional Care Evaluation involves the promotion and maintenance of high quality care, through the analysis, review and evaluation of the clinical practice that exists within the hospital. To accomplish such analysis effectively, criteria for evaluating professional care must be established by the medical staff. Findings relative to professional care evaluation should be compared with the criteria established by the medical staff. The means of carrying out a continuous program of clinical care surveillance is left to the individual hospital. There must be evidence that the major clinical activities of the hospital are under regular surveillance, and that the results are being utilized to further medical education and to improve patterns of care, for the hospital to be eligible for accreditation status after January, 1977."

The Guide to Hospital Accreditation states:

"The essential characteristics of an acceptable patient care evaluation process are:

1. Criteria of optimal achievable care, set by the hospital's own medical staff, must be measurable, with emphasis on justification for medical intervention and on patient outcomes.

2. Comparison of actual clinical practices against these predetermined criteria must take place.

3. Results must be analyzed by means of peer review. Clinically valid, acceptable variations must be separated from those that cannot be justified.

4. Action must be taken on variations deemed not justified.

5. Follow-up must occur after an appropriate interval to make sure action has been taken and has resulted in correction of any problems identified.

6. Documented reports of the results of all audit activities must go to the appropriate clinical departments, the medical advisory committee, the chief of the medical staff and to the hospital's governing body."

In a presentation at a C.C.H.A. workshop on patient care appraisal, Murray (2) noted that, in spite of trying to avoid giving a stamp of approval to any one system of appraisal, the term "criteria" has been interpreted, not in its generic sense, as was intended, but as support for a single form of patient care appraisal, a misapprehension that will require time and experience with the accreditation process to correct. Murray (2) also cited data from an analysis of the results of accreditation surveys carried out during 1978:

> 38% of the hospitals surveyed received an accreditation award for 3 years, indicating that they had regular on-going professional care evaluation programs in effect. Another 55% ... had at least made some start on structured studies and so achieved the rating of Accreditation for 2 years.

It was concluded that the degree of voluntary compliance with the new standards was "very satisfying."

Psychiatric Services

Between 1972 and 1978 the J.C.A.H. and the C.C.H.A. developed divergent approaches to the setting of standards for psychiatric facilities. One of the major differences lay in a decision of the C.C.H.A. to avoid developing sets of standards for each sub-type of facility, e.g. child,adolescent, or alcoholism and drug abuse facilities, believing that the principles of the accreditation process could be applied to a broad range of health facilities. The J.C.A.H., on the other hand, developed separate sets of standards for several types of facilities. In this instance, the Canadian approach has become the model for both accrediting bodies. The J.C.A.H. has just published the "Consolidated Standards for Child, Adolescent and Adult Psychiatric, Alcoholism and Drug Abuse Programs" (4).

While compliance with Standard V is a "must" for general hospitals, in order to receive full 3-year Accreditation, the Canadian Council has decided that the state of the art of patient care appraisal in psychiatric facilities has not reached a level that would warrant making Standard V a prerequisite for full Accreditation status.

In a recent memorandum to all accredited hospitals (5) the Executive Director of the C.C.H.A. made the following statement: "C.C.H.A. does not have specific guidelines for clinical appraisal in mental health services or long-term care centres. Mental Health Services and Long Term Centres are strongly encouraged to develop appropriate systems."

In a paper presented at the annual meeting of the Canadian Psychiatric Association in Halifax in 1978, Awad et al (6) reported on the findings of a survey of psychiatric facilities--hospitals and general hospital units--in Ontario, which was aimed at ascertaining the current status of audits of the quality of patient care. The findings indicated that all but one of the provincially operated psychiatric hospitals were using some type of formal audit procedure, as opposed to 65% of responding general hospital psychiatric units, 45% of private, semi-private, and community psychiatric hospitals, and 40% of children's psychiatric and mental retardation facilities. 52% of the responding facilities reported using comprehensive audits (covering all aspects of patient care) rather than limiting audits to specific treatment modalities, suicide reviews, etc. 64% of audits were developed and carried out on a multidisciplinary basis. 50% of the respondents reported that, in their opinion, audits had contributed to improvement in psychiatric care, and 71% felt that audits had contributed to favorable developments in the area of continuing staff education.

In 1976 the Accreditation Council for Psychiatric Facilities (AC/PF) of the U.S. Joint Commission adopted a new patient care audit Standard entitled "Quality of Professional Services," which was to apply to all facilities seeking AC/PF accreditation as of July 1, 1977. Quantitatively this meant that facilities and programs seeking AC/PF accreditation would have to demonstrate that they had developed, or were in the process of developing, a system that met audit standards, and that by July 1977 every facility should have two audits in progress (topics selected and audit criteria established). As in Canada, minimal levels were used because of the relative inexperience with audits of patient care in mental health facilities. To correct this situation, the J.C.A.H.'s Quality Resource Centre and the AC/PF set up Psychiatric Audit Team Seminars (PATS) to help mental health facility staff and program staff develop the skills required to meet the new Standard.

As noted above, the C.C.H.A. does not yet feel that a similar Standard can be made mandatory for Canadian psychiatric facilities and programs.

Other Approaches

Canadian medical organizations other than the C.C.H.A. have independently endorsed clinical care appraisal systems. These reflect the concerns of organized medicine, including psychiatry. The Canadian Medical Association in 1976 resolved that "the C.M.A. seek ways of developing the capabilities for providing expertise to assist the Divisions (of the C.M.A.) in physician-initiated patient care appraisal programs for both ambulatory and hospital care." The Canadian Psychiatric Association has established a Task Force on Peer Review to study the application of patient care appraisal methods to mental health services, and the C.P.A. Council on Education and Professional Liaison was commissioned in 1978 to undertake a detailed, Canada-wide study of "patient care review procedures" (7). The Ontario Psychiatric Association has directed its attention to a method of patient care appraisal, the consultation audit model, that could be used by those engaged primarily in private practice (8). The Ontario Psychiatric Hospitals and Hospital Schools Medical Staff Association has recently published a set of "Recommendations on Peer Review" (9).

In the United States, the expansion of federally funded health insurance programs like Medicare and Medicaid, and the concerns about the quality of care and cost containment have led to the establishment, by law, of Professional Standards Review Organizations (P.S.R.O.'s). This approach, which involves utilization review, medical audit, and project monitoring, has had mixed results (10, 11), but will undoubtedly be a feature of the U. S. scene for some years to come.

Problems

1) Validation

Patient care appraisal has its own inherent difficulties. These include the "so what" response of those who see evaluation of quality of care and peer review as expensive, time-consuming, and unrelated in any demonstrable way to actual improvement in the quality of patient care.

Tugwell (12), in a presentation to a meeting of C.C.H.A. surveyors, underlined several important limitations of process evaluation: "the Standards against which the performance is judged are usually not based on clinical outcome but upon what is considered to be good practice by leaders of the profession; validation of such process strategies against outcome has had to await the development of feasible and valid outcome measures; the cost of both the implementation of the process strategies and of rectifying the deficiencies identified is considerable; current process strategies fail to include assessment of important dimensions of care such as patient education."

2) Methodology

Brook (1) states that the major difficulties in quality assessment are related to methodology: reliance on the medical record as the source of data, the use of process rather than outcome criteria, and failure to use decision analysis methods in establishing criteria. He recommends that research concentrate on developing valid measures of the quality of what he terms the "art-of-care" (the milieu, manner, and behavior of the provider in delivering the care to, and communicating with, the patient), as opposed to "technical care" (diagnostic and therapeutic processes). Like the C.C.H.A., which sees quality assurance as an on-going evolutionary process, Brook warns against attempting to develop an ideal system in the next few years unless carefully evaluated research is carried out which would lead to the elimination of quality assurance activities that do not improve health status, and the retention and expansion of only those that do.

Green (12) states that an "optimal care" approach tends to include as many procedures as possible that might be consistent with a given diagnosis, "undoubtedly fostered by the fear that, with the advent of PSRO's, reimbursement might be denied for any procedure not so listed." Such "laundry lists" become unwieldy, meaningless, and irrelevant for specific cases and do not allow discrimination as to the quality of care provided. The use of 'validated criteria' has been recommended as a more useful alternative (18).

3) Medicolegal Aspects

In the same surveyors' conference mentioned above, three medicolegal hazards of patient care appraisal were reviewed (13):

a) liability of the members of an audit committee to action for libel or slander as a result of their written or spoken reports concerning the level of practice of individual members of the medical staff. It was noted that such liability has been foreseen, and almost all Canadian provinces have provided statutory immunity for members acting in good faith.

b) use of agreed-upon criteria for acceptable levels of practice in the hospital as minimum criteria for acceptable practice, thus making non-compliance tantamount to proof of malpractice. While not very reassuring, it was noted that such use of accepted criteria for desirable patterns of practice has not yet occurred in Canada (although it has occurred in the United States). It was strongly recommended that terms such as 'guidelines' should be used to designate desirable criteria for optimal practice, rather than implying mandatory minimums.

c) subpoena by a patient's lawyer of audit worksheets, to be used to indicate that the doctor in question had come to the attention of the audit committee more frequently than his colleagues. It was noted that tissue committee records have been available for over 30 years. While such action is certainly possible, again it has yet to occur in Canada. As a remedy, it was suggested that worksheets need not be retained, but only summaries and narrative reports.

CANADA-U.S. DIFFERENCES AND SIMILARITIES

Spiralling costs of health care, third party payers, faltering economies and consumer pressures in both Canada and the United States have intensified professional concerns about the quality of health care services. However, there are significant differences between our two countries in the evaluation of health care. Kent and Nicholls (14) have noted that "the pressures favoring an evolution in Canada similar to that in the United States have not yet become so powerful or so urgent as to compel a hasty and perhaps ill-judged adoption of measures which have yet to prove their efficacy in the United States."

In a review of "Quality Assurance Strategies in U.S. and Canadian Psychiatry", Firth (15) notes that the traditional structural approach of hospital accreditation surveys is an indirect approach of limited value. However, he does point out that "the recent Canadian accreditation 'requirement' of hospitals to demonstrate evaluation systems suggests a more dynamic role than simply assuring a 'house in order'. Chronologically, this shift occurred when the Joint Commission's Accreditation Council for Psychiatric Facilities established a stricter audit standard.

Firth concludes that "because of the very different health and social systems much [of the U.S. approach] is not useful or relevant to the Canadian situation . . . [and] because mechanisms exist in Canada to contain costs [e.g. provincial government control of hospital budgets and the monitoring of physician practice profiles], perhaps more emphasis can be placed by the profession on quality assurance . . . that is, developing techniques of improving demonstrated deficiencies . . . whatever systems are developed here [in Canada] they should have built-in means of self-assessment, so that the important question is not left begging: namely, do quality assurance strategies assure quality?"

Summary

The Canadian Council on Hospital Accreditation and the American Joint Commission on Accreditation of Hospitals have, since their establishment, supported and promoted the development of procedures to evaluate the quality of patient care provided in health facilities. Although originally almost exclusively concerned with structural criteria, both accrediting bodies have, particularly in the last decade, increasingly emphasized the process aspects of quality of care appraisal. Since 1977 both the C.C.H.A. and the J.C.A.H. have required evidence of on-going internal surveillance of the major clinical activities of each hospital being surveyed before awarding full Accreditation status. While psychiatric facilities are strongly encouraged to develop appropriate means for quality of care appraisal, the C.C.H.A. does not believe that the 'state of the art' has yet reached the point where full-scale audits can be made a prerequisite for full accreditation.

REFERENCES

1. Brook, P.H., Quality Assurance Mechanisms in the United States: from there to where? Question of Quality - Road to Assurance in Medical Care. Chapt. 12. Ed. G. McLachlan. Oxford University Press, (1976).

2. Murray, J.A., Patient Care Appraisal Workshop - C.C.H.A. Requirements. Presented at Vancouver General Hospital, (1979).

3. Guide to Hospital Accreditation 1977, Canadian Council on Hospital Accreditation, (1977).

4. Joint Commission on Accreditation of Hospitals, J.C.A.H. Standards for Child, Adolescent and Adult Psychiatry, Alcoholism and Drug Abuse Programs. Chicago, Illinois, (1979).

5. Swanson, A.L., Memorandum to all C.C.H.A. Accredited Hospitals. Subject: CCHA Requirements for Clinical Appraisal (Medical Audit), (1978).

6. Awad, A., Durost, H., Gray, J., Kugelmass, M., Smith, C., Psychiatric Audits - the Ontario Scene. Can. J. Psychiatry, in press.

7. Thompson, M.G.C., Questionnaire in Patient Care Review Procedures. Council on Education and Professional Liaison: Canadian Psychiatric Association, (1978).

8. Raschka, L.B., Annual Report, Committee on Peer Review and Continuing Medical Education: Ontario Psychiatric Association, (1978).

9. Awad, A.G., Bardhan, B., Crane, H.G., Galbraith, D.A., Peer Review, Ontario Psychiatric Hospitals and Hospital Schools Medical Staff Association, (1979).

10. Langley, D.G., Peer Review, Prospects and Problems: Am. J. Psychiatry, 130:301-304, (1973).

11. Anderson, O.W., PSRO's, the Medical Profession and the Public Interest. Milbank Mem. Fund Quart./Health and Society: 379-388, (1976).

12. Green, R., Assessing the Quality of Care - the State of the Art. Cambridge, Bellinger Co., (1976).

13. Tugwell, P., Review of Process Measurement of Quality of Care. Presented at Annual C.C.H.A. Surveyors Conference, Toronto, (1979).

14. Murray, J. A., Summary Report on Medico-Legal Hazards of Patient Care Appraisal. Presented at Annual C.C.H.A. Surveyors Conference, Toronto, (1979).

15. Kent, I., Nicholls, W., Peer Review for Canada. Can. Psychiat. Assoc. J., 22: 49-56, (1977).

16. Firth, J., Quality Assurance Strategies in U. S. and Canadian Psychiatry. Can. J. Psychiatry, 24: 309-315, (1979).

Peer Review and the Use of Psychotropic Drugs

Richard Dorsey, M.D.

Why the APA Developed Screening Criteria

This paper will discuss the American Psychiatric Association's screening criteria for psychotropic drug use, what lay behind that project, and how it may be useful in Canada.

Psychotropic drugs are among the most widely prescribed class of drugs in all of medicine. They are probably the leading tool in psychiatry, and are commonly used in other specialities as well. For example, diazepam has been the most widely prescribed drug in many western countries, and as a class the benzodiazepines rank with antibiotics and anti-hypertensive drugs in utilization.

For this reason we took great care to develop a set of screening criteria that would apply not only to psychiatrists or to the kinds of patients that psychiatrists treat, but which could be used to monitor the prescribing of physicians in many specialities. This was done in part to broaden the utility of the criteria, but also was in keeping with a basic philosophical decision that organized medicine has taken in the United States: to emphasize the right of the physician to treat particular kinds of patients as long as he does it well, without regard to speciality qualification. We have chosen to avoid what we believe was a mistake in the United Kingdom thirty years ago, when physicians were polarized into specialists against generalists. For both medical and political reasons we have tried to maintain as much cohesion as possible, and this is reflected in the kind of criteria we have developed.

Clearly, there are several reasons for reviewing the prescribing of drugs in general, and of psychotropic drugs in particular. One is *medical quality*. Some studies suggest that physicians, including psychiatrists, have less expertise in the use of psychotropic drugs than other specialists have in the use of drugs in their fields. That is, cardiologists tend to know more about digitalis or diuretics than psychiatrists as a group know about antipsychotic drugs. This is partly due to the division we have had in psychiatry between the psychotherapists, who have used drugs somewhat sparingly, and the biologic psychiatrists, whose main interest has always been in the use of medications. Outside psychiatry, despite the fact that a large proportion of his patients have mental disorders, the average doctor tends to be quite uncomfortable with his own knowledge when prescribing anything beyond benzodiazepines and the sedative hypnotic drugs.

The second reason for review is *medical necessity*. In insurance contracts in the United States medical necessity has a very specific meaning: "pay or no pay". If something is medically necessary, the patient pays. One aspect of this, whether money should be paid for drugs that are not given for proper indications, has been a problem for psychiatry. One group argues in essence that a little mental suffering builds character, and that prescribing drugs for what really ought to be part of a growth experience not only is bad medicine, but bad morals as well. Many of the people who hold this view have never had mental illness themselves, nor seen it in their relatives, nor dealt with it first hand.

A third reason for reviewing the prescribing of drugs is *political accountability*, as government--either directly through paying the bills, or indirectly through regulatory and legal processes--takes a major role in the practice of medicine. In the United States we have a federal program for the aged, Medicare, and one for the indigent, Medicaid. A substantial share of all expenses for health care is provided by the government, which, as the budgets get tighter, wants to know what it is buying. Governments are not content for physicians to simply offer general verbal reassurance that the government is getting its money's worth. It should be mentioned that political accountability has been accompanied by the setting of standards to some extent as an end in itself. Governments write regulations, and the people who go into government administration are fond of that kind of activity. Just as doctors like to prescribe and surgeons like to operate, regulators like to regulate, and given a chance to do so, they will.

Finally, there is the problem of the *involuntarily committed patient*, a patient deprived in some jurisdictions of the freedom to choose whether to be treated or not. We need to assure both the public and the courts that the patient treated against his will is receiving the proper medication. Screening criteria for drugs are a step towards this assurance.

The American Psychiatric Association was spurred into writing criteria partly because several of our states were developing "guidelines" which were, in effect, "cookbooks" telling doctors how they shoud be using drugs. These guidelines did not address our major concern: isolating deviant cases through screening processes. In addition, many of these guidelines were written by people with relatively limited clinical experience, who tended to greatly over-simplify the practice of medicine by saying that because something should be done 80 percent of the time, it should be done *all* of the time. Actually, it is relatively easy to write a standard for what should be done half of the time, but the closer you get to a standard which applies to all cases, the more difficult the exercise becomes and the broader and more vague the criteria.

We did not want to see such "guidelines" imposed on psychiatrists in either the public or the private sector. In one state, the federal courts in essence took the state hospital system into receivership, and required that physicians prescribe only according to drug labelling. Drug labelling is useful as a constraint on pharmaceutical promotion, and as a source of information, but it should certainly not be taken as a definition of optimal care for a deviant population. We saw clearly, however, that this trend would continue unless we took some action to pre-empt it. We also correctly anticipated what did happen to our surgical colleagues--that politicians would turn so-called inappropriate psychotropic prescribing into a political issue.

Since we developed our criteria in advance of major governmental regulations, we have so far stayed out of difficulty. Our surgical colleagues, on the other hand, could not believe that anyone would ever question something as tangible as an operation, and, to their sorrow, have found themselves saddled with second opinion programs and the need to write criteria under considerable time pressure and public pressure.

How the APA Developed Screening Criteria

The process we went through in developing our screening criteria may be helpful to Canadian psychiatrists in formulating psychotropic criteria for any other kind of review. We began by contracting with one of the scientific agencies of our Government, the National Institute of Mental Health, rather than with one of the regulatory agencies such as the Health Care Financing Administration or the Food and Drug Administration. We think this is a critical difference, not only in terms of the kind of work we will be able to do, but in terms of how the practitioner perceives the system that will ultimately review his work.

Our task force, the people who actually wrote the criteria, were all expert psychopharmacologists with some knowledge of peer review. Government has an unfortunate tendency to stop here: to get experts to do something and then try to apply their results to generalists without any intermediate steps. To some extent hospitals and insurers share the same tendency. After the experts had developed the criteria, we had them reviewed by generalists--first members of APA's Peer Review Committee, and then the elected leaders of the American Psychiatric Association--to determine whether the criteria were genuinely applicable to general psychiatric practice. We then went a step further, and circulated the criteria among the American Medical Association, the American College of Physicians (internal medicine specialists), and the American Academy of Family Physicians (family practitioners). We did not submit a final draft to the government until each of these organizations was satisfied with the criteria and regarded them as valid for medical practice generally.

Finally, we published them, not in a psychiatric journal, but in the Journal of the American Medical Association, in order to reach general physicians.

The Criteria

This section will briefly discuss the philosophy behind the screening criteria, define several terms contained in them, and describe how to use the criteria in case reviews. It will be helpful to the reader to refer to the "Psychopharmacological Screening Criteria" (Appendix A, p. 57-74) during this discussion.

Purpose and Philosophy

In our first publication on this subject (1) we explicitly stated that we were developing screening criteria to allow a nurse to select from a large number of cases a small number which were deviant. We made the distinction between an exception and a deficiency: exception means deviant only in a statistical sense. In many cases also, the reason for the supposed deviance is medical necessity or good medical judgement. We also made the distinction between optimal practice and acceptable practice. There is a strong temptation among reviewers to say that anything less than optimal is unacceptable. That mistake can lead to sacrificing something good for unattainable perfection. Furthermore, the best experts disagree, and even where they agree, optimal by definition means "the best that can be done." Realistically, all doctors cannot be expected to practice the best medicine, any more than all governors can be expected to be the greatest statesmen or all lawyers to be the greatest barristers. In general, it is much wiser to weed out very bad practice, than to try to say that anything less than perfection is unacceptable.

One of our main criteria for acceptable practice was general documentation in every patient's chart. For example, if a patient were taking a psychotropic drug without having had a mental status examination, this would be a reviewable case no matter what the drug. We then looked at specific drug classes and designed criteria appropriate to each class.

The decision of the physician reviewers is based on the record. Rarely do they actually interview the patient--only if there is a strong suspicion of fraud or abuse, or a great discrepancy between what the doctor has recorded and other kinds of evidence. Otherwise, we assume that the record itself is sufficient and accurate. This means that the doctor must include enough information in patients' charts to permit another doctor to examine them and reach some conclusion. We have been able to get most of our colleagues to do this.

We also felt that minimal documentation should be present in the outpatient record. While we recognized that there are differences in record-keeping between outpatient clinics and private doctors' offices, we felt that when the government or a third party begins paying for medications, outpatient records will be important to physicians in answering such questions as: "Is there a history, physical examination, and mental status examination?"

A lot of controversy exists in North American psychiatry as to who should get psychotherapy, who should get antidepressant medications, and who should get both. Very respected physicians have argued on both sides of this issue. Our view has been that as a reasonable number of doctors are treating patients in a particular way, the doctor being reviewed who has prescribed according to such current practice satisfies the criteria, even though the physician reviewer might have treated the patient differently. Thus, the reviewer must not only understand his own practice, but must also know something about the range of practice in his community.

Format

The importance we placed on documentation is reflected in the first two sections of the criteria (Appendix A,pp. 57, 58). Most other topics are similarly divided into inpatient and outpatient sections, indicating the different circumstances in each situation, yet also the importance of standards and record-keeping in each.

All sections are organized according to a system of "review if [the item is] absent" or "review if present." There are other ways of organizing the criteria, but we think this is the clearest. It simply tells the reader that if, for example, item A is absent, this chart should be pulled out for review.

Discussion of Selected Terms: Inpatient and Outpatient Documentation (p. 57)

"Mental status examination" touches on the issue of optimal criteria. In several areas we felt that diagnostic procedures were less than adequate. Instead of demanding that all doctors in North America conform to our standards, which would have been presumptuous and provocative, we recommended that the reviewing organization at least consider applying the criterion of a mental status examination. For example, the non-psychiatric physician who is prescribing an antianxiety drug should have some note on the record indicating what mental symptoms are present and on what diagnosis he has based his choice of therapy.

Several other itmes under B--"Minimal documentation"--apply more to the public sector than to the private, but we think that any physician who treats patients, or anyone else who acts as primary therapist under the supervision of a physician, should provide the kind of information listed (history, physical exam, physician diagnosis, treatment plan, etc.)

The criterion "generally accepted dosage range" indicates that if a particular patient is getting more than or less than the usual dose, the chart should be pulled out for review. The doctor is not obliged to prescribe any particular dose, but where there is deviant dosage, another physician should take a look.

"Unusual duration of therapy" suggests looking at the short end as well as the long end, particularly on inpatient services. If a patient is given a drug for only two days, two questions arise: whether the drug should have been prescribed at all, and whether it was given a fair trial. Problems with concomitant medications depend upon the particular drugs given; including the criterion may help alert doctors to harmful interactions.

"Critical adverse developments," such as tardive dyskinesia in a patient on antipsychotic drugs, call for a review to see whether the doctor is aware that the adverse effect has occurred, has made the connection between the adverse effect and the drug, and has taken reasonable action to minimize or correct it. "Critical adjunctive services" refer to other forms of treatment the patient may need if a particular kind of medication is being used. Finally, we used the qualifier "relative" with "contraindications" to emphasize that few things in psychiatry or in medicine are always contraindicated. Contraindication generally means that there is a very high risk, but in a specific case the doctor may have a good reason for taking this risk, or may feel that for a particular patient, the level of risk is acceptable.

Discussion of Selected Terms: Medication Criteria Sets

We will now consider some specific criteria sets. *Antianxiety medications* (p.58) are commonly indicated for anxiety associated with neuroses, psychophysiological disorders, physical illness and injury, alcoholism, and alcohol withdrawal.

If one of these diagnoses is present in the chart, there is no need to review that case for appropriateness of drug selection. If one of these diagnoses is not present, the case goes out to physician review. There may be other grounds for having used an antianxiety drug, but these diagnoses are the leading ones.

Minimal documentation requires history, physical examination, and mental status exam. Dosage ranges represent common usage, not the extremes.

If the duration of medication is less than three days, we should ask "Was it a fair trial?" and "Was it necessary in the first place?" Frequent changes in drugs suggest that the doctor may not be persevering long enough, or perhaps is jumping and guessing. Because this class of drugs is generally not used for lifetime maintenance, at the end of three months the doctor should determine whether the patient still needs the medication, and if so, why.

Giving two benzodiazepines at once makes relatively little sense. However, we sometimes find a patient who is seeing several doctors; one may be giving the patient oxazepam, another may be prescribing diazepam and a third flurazepam.

In very few cases, using antipsychotic drugs along with antianxiety drugs may be useful, but the first question we should ask is whether the patient was given a sufficient dose of antipsychotic drug in the first place. Polypharmacy--the use of small doses of many drugs rather than adequate doses of fewer--is a major problem in psychopharmacology, and is receiving increased attention in physician review.

"Adverse developments" include no improvement, unusual length of stay in hospital, sedation and lethargy, and ataxia. Some of these criteria are designed primarily to alert the physician.

Delirium, confusion, and intentional overdose raise the question of whether the patient was in fact depressed rather than suffering primarily from an anxiety syndrome. Withdrawal symptoms on discontinuation suggest that the patient may have taken too much for too long.

Antipsychotic medications are broken down into psychotic and non-psychotic disorders and subdivided further to inpatient and outpatient sets. The first such set--"Antipsychotic Medications (Psychotic Disorders) Inpatient Criteria" (p. 61)--will serve as an example. The common indications (schizophrenia, organic brain syndrome, manic depressive illness in a psychotic state) no one argues about at all. We were able to get a majority, but not unanimity even among ourselves, on the two other indications (psychotic depressive reaction and manic depressive illness, depressed type). However, all of us recognized that these conditions were widely treated with antipsychotic drugs, and that to recommend that all those cases be pulled for review would not be appropriate.

Giving more than one antipsychotic drug at a time is generally regarded as irrational therapy. There may occasionally be a reason for it, but the burden should be on the prescriber to set forth that reason. A frequent problem occurs when antipsychotic drugs are used with anticholinergic drugs for functional GI syndromes. Patients may experience toxic psychoses, urinary difficulty, or constipation. The doctor may not recognize these as side effects, and may consequently prescribe more medication rather than less.

Common side effects of the antipsychotic drugs include persistent sedation, urinary retention, and syncope. Death--whether drug related or not--occurs infrequently; it is always worth investigating *why* a psychiatric patient dies. Tardive dyskinesia should be considered, as should significant abnormalities in laboratory tests if they occur.

For adjunctive services a patient should have basic laboratory studies on admission. We recommend ECG's for patients over 65 or if there is a history of cardiac disorder. Different parts of United States or Canada might set different age limits--perhaps 40 instead of 65; it is easy enough to change the numbers if there is a basic framework.

Relative contraindications for antipsychotic drugs include allergy to drug, recent myocardial infarction, previous tardive dyskinesia, or a very young patient.

In outpatient criteria for the same class of drugs, the only real difference is that the recommended doses are relatively lower than for inpatients, reflecting prevailing practice.

The "Fixed-Radio Combination Products" criteria (p.66) represented a real difference of opinion between the group of experts and what we recognized to be prevailing practice. I think if it were our decision, we probably would not have fixed ratio combination products in the first place, but they meet the

American and Canadian legal standards for being sold (i.e., they were shown to be safe and effective at the time that they were initially marketed) and are still widely used. In our country, a fixed ratio combination of amitriptyline and perphenazine is the most widely used drug for depression.

Applying the Criteria in Canada and the United States

In conclusion, there are several possible applications for these criteria in Canada or the United States. One is reviewing quality; a trade-off between cost and quality may not be inevitable, particularly in psychiatry. There is a book circulating in business circles in the United States called "Quality is Free", whose central thesis is that so much money is saved by doing something right the first time, that whatever it costs is worth it. I think that in terms of saving hospital time, health care personnel time, patient morbidity, social insurance payments and so on, using these drugs optimally is worth a substantially heavier investment in education, in review, and in quality assurance than is now being made.

The criteria could certainly be used to audit existing programs. For example, the National Institute of Mental Health in the United States funds many community mental health centers, and intends to use the criteria for reviewing these facilities.

The criteria can also be used for general quality or medical care evaluation studies. In hospitals where staffs are spread thin and many doctors are not fully trained in psychiatry, the criteria are being used to monitor performance, with the pharmacist deciding when to ask a senior physician to check a particular prescription. Many doctors would not like to practice under those circumstances. The senior doctors, however, find much merit in being aware of unusual prescribing practices when they are occurring, rather than a year later. If there is a problem, they can correct it for the patient's benefit, and equally important, they can talk with the attending doctor and do their educating immediately.

We also hope that these criteria can be used for educating practitioners in general. Simply by reading the criteria, physicians involved in treatment and review may gain specific knowledge in, and a broader perspective of, the use of psychotropic drugs.

Drug therapy has significantly changed the treatment of the mentally ill. We feel that as more new drugs become available, a review of drug prescribing becomes even more necessary, and that, in addition, this kind of review will naturally grow as medical practice review grows generally.

We hope that our work will make it easier to review the quality of psychotropic prescribing, and to do it in a way this is clinically relevant.

REFERENCES

1. Dorsey, R., Ayd, F.J., Cole, J., Klein, D., Simpson, G., Tupin, J., DiMascio, A., Psychopharmacological Screening Criteria Development Project, JAMA 241, 10 (1979).

APPENDIX A*

Psychopharmacological Criteria: Inpatient Documentation

Review If:

Absent A. Common professionally accepted indications (should account for approximately 90% of use)

Absent B. Minimal documentation (should be present in at least 90% of charts)
1. History
2. Physical examination
3. Mental status examination (optional on nonpsychiatric services)
4. Diagnosis made or approved by physician
5. Treatment plan developed or approved by physician
6. Medication order signed by physician
7. Progress notes made and signed by physician at intervals not greater than three days
8. Nurses' notes, daily recording of
   a. Drug administration as ordered by physician
   b. General clinical observations
9. Graphical record, including
   a. Vital signs (temperature, pulse, respiration, blood pressure) at least once daily
   b. Other observations as ordered by physician
10. Laboratory reports (including roentgenogram and ECG) as ordered by physician
11. Discharge summary if patient has left hospital at the time review occurs

Review If:

Absent C. Generally accepted dosage range (should apply to approximately 90% of patients)

Present D. Unusual duration of therapy (should occur in less than 10% of patients)

E. Unusual concomitant prescribing
1. Psychotropic medications
2. Other medications

Present F. Critical adverse developments

Absent G. Critical adjunctive services

Present H. Relative contraindications

---

* For Canadian trade names of drugs mentioned see p.75.

Psychopharmacologic Criteria: Outpatient Documentation

Review If:

Absent A. Common professionally accepted indications (should account for approximately 90% of use)

B. Minimal documentation (should be present in at least 90% of charts)
1. History
2. Physical examination at time of initial interview or within last six months
3. Mental status examination (optional on non-psychiatric services)
4. Diagnosis made or approved by physician
5. Treatment plan approved or developed by physician
6. Record of medication prescribed by physician
7. Progress note by primary therapist on each patient visit; progress note by physician at least once every three months
8. Record of administration of any injection as ordered by physician
9. Laboratory reports (including roentgenogram and ECT) as ordered by physician

Absent C. Generally accepted dosage range (should apply to approximately 90% of patients)

Present D. Unusual duration of therapy (should occur in less than 10% of patients)

Present E. Unusual concomitant prescribing
1. Psychotropic medications
2. Other medications

Present F. Critical adverse developments

Absent G. Critical adjunctive services

Present H. Relative contraindications

Antianxiety Medications: Inpatient and Outpatient Criteria

Review If:

Absent A. Common indications (validate by AMA and Department of Health, Education, and Welfare [DHEW] criteria if desired)
1. Anxiety associated with neuroses
2. Anxiety associated with psychophysiological disorders
3. Anxiety associated with physical illness or injury
4. Anxiety associated with alcoholism or alcohol withdrawal

Absent B. Minimal documentation (all standard inpatient or outpatient requirements)

Absent C. Dosage range, mg/day

	Generic	Trade Names (for Canadian Trade Names see p. 75)	Younger Than 65 Years	Older Than 65 and Younger Than 12 Years
1.	Chlordiazepoxide hydrochloride	Chlordiazachel Caps, Librium, SKF-Lygen	20-100	10.0-40
2.	Diazepam	Valium	10-60	2.5-20
3.	Oxazepam	Serax	15-90	10.0-60
4.	Clorazepate dipotassium	Tranxene	15-60	7.5-30
5.	Prazepam	Verstran	20-60	10.0-30
6.	Lorazepam	Ativan	2-6	0.5-3
7.	Meprobamate	Equanil, Miltown	400-1,600	200.0-600

Present D. Duration
1. Less than three days
2. More than two changes of psychotropic medication in any seven-day period
3. Benzodiazepine more than three months
4. Meprobamate more than two months

Review If:
Present E. Concomitance
1. Any other benzodiazepine (except flurazepam hydrochloride)
2. Any antipsychotic drug for the aforementioned indications
3. More than one other psychotropic medication of any class

Present F. Critical adverse development
1. No improvement by local 60th percentile length of stay (LOS) for diagnosis (or seven days)
2. Patient still in hospital by local 90th percentile LOS for diagnosis (or 14 days)
3. Marked sedation or lethargy after the first week
4. Ataxia (especially in the elderly)
5. Delirium or confusion
6. Intentional overdose
7. Withdrawal symptoms on discontinuation of therapy

Absent G. Critical adjunctive services
1. Basic laboratory studies on admission

Present H. Relative contraindications
1. History of allergy to this drug
2. Age younger than 5 years

Antiparkinsonism Medication (Except Levodopa): Inpatient and Outpatient Criteria

Review If:

Absent A. Common indications
1. Treatment of Parkinson's disease
2. Alleviation of extrapyramidal side effects (EPSEs) induced by antipsychotic drugs
3. Use in prophylaxis of EPSE induced by antipsychotic drugs (optional criterion)

Absent B. Minimal documentation (all standard inpatient or outpatient requirements)
1. Should include statement that patient has EPSE after antipsychotic drug therapy was initiated or that patient has symptoms of Parkinson's disease

Absent C. Dosage range, mg

	For EPSE	For Parkinson's Disease
1. Amantadine hydrochloride (Symmetrel)	100-200	100.0-400
2. Benztropine mesylate (Cogentin Mesylate)	1-8	0.5-6
3. Biperiden hydrochloride (Akineton Hydrochloride)	2-8	4.0-8
4. Diphenhydramine hydrochloride (Benadryl)	50-150	50.0-300
5. Procyclidine hydrochloride (Kemadrin)	6-20	6.0-25
6. Trihexyphenidyl hydrochloride (Antitrem, Artane, Pipanol, Tremin Hydrochloride)	1-10	2.0-15

Present D. Duration
1. More than four months, except for Parkinson's disease

Review If:

Present E. Concomitance
1. Any antidepressant
2. Any other anticholingergic medication (except an antipsychotic)
3. For diphenhydramine only, any MAO inhibitor

Present F. Critical adverse developments
1. Urinary retention
2. Severe constipation
3. Delirium

Absent G. Critical adjunctive services (inpatient only)
1. Basic laboratory studies on admission
2. Daily vital signs for patients older than 65 years of age

Present H. Relative contraindications
1. History of allergy to this class of drugs
2. Angle closure glaucoma (except for amantadine)
3. Prostatic hypertrophy (except for amantadine)
4. Tardive dyskinesia
5. Age younger than 5 years

Antipsychotic Medications (Psychotic Disorders): Inpatient Criteria

Review If:

Absent A. Common indications (validate by AMA/DHEW criteria if desired)
1. Schizophrenia, any subtype
2. Organic brain syndrome with psychosis
3. Manic-depressive illness (manic and circular)
4. Psychotic depressive reaction (optional criterion)
5. Manic-depressive illness, depressed (optional criterion)

Absent B. Minimal documentation (all standard inpatient requirements)

C. Dosage range (chlorpromazine equivalents)
1. Patients aged 13 to 64 years 200 to 1,600 mg daily (200 to 800 mg for thioridazine)
2. Patients aged 65 years or older (except organic brain syndrome): 100 to 800 mg daily (one half usual adult dose)
3. Patients aged 65 years or older (with organic brain syndrome): 50 to 400 mg daily (one fourth usual adult dose)
4. Patients aged 5 to 12 years: 50 to 400 mg daily (one fourth usual adult dose)

Present D. Duration
1. Less than three days
2. More than two changes of psychotropic medication in any seven-day period

Review If:

Present E. Concomitance
1. Any other antipsychotic drug
2. More than one other psychotropic drug of any class
3. Anticholinergic or antispasmodic gastrointestinal (GI) medications

Present F. Critical adverse developments
1. No improvement by 60th percentile LOS for diagnosis (or 21st day)
2. Patient still in hospital by 90th percentile LOS for diagnosis (or 28th day)
3. Marked sedation or lethargy after one week
4. Urinary retention
5. Syncope

6. Convulsion
7. Death from any cause
8. Tardive dyskinesia
9. Any follow-up laboratory abnormalities during treatment, e.g.
   a. Bilirubin level greater than 1.0 mg/dl
   b. SGOT level greater than 100 IU/ml
   c. WBC count less than 3,000/cu mm

Absent G. Critical adjunctive services
1. Basic laboratory studies on admission
2. ECG on admission for patients older than 65 years of age or history of cardiac disorder

Present H. Relative contraindications
1. History of allergy to this drug
2. Myocardial infarction within six weeks
3. History of tardive dyskinesia
4. Age younger than 5 years

Antipsychotic Medications (Psychotic Disorders): Outpatient Criteria

Review If:

Absent A. Common indications (validate by AMA/DHEW criteria if desired)
1. Schizophrenia, any subtype
2. Organic brain syndrome with psychosis
3. Manic-depressive illness (manic and circular
4. Involutional melancholia (optional criterion)
5. Psychotic depressive reaction (optional criterion)
6. Childhood psychosis

Absent B. Minimal documentation (all standard outpatient requirements), plus note every three months about presence or absence of tardive dyskinesia

Absent C. Dosage range (chlorpromazine equivalents)
1. Patients aged 13 to 64 years: 50 to 800 mg equivalent daily
2. Patients aged 65 years or older (except organic brain syndrome): 25 to 400 mg daily (one half usual adult dose)
3. Patients aged 65 years or older (organic brain syndrome): 10 to 200 mg daily (one fourth usual adult dose)
4. Patients aged 5 to 12 years: 10 to 200 mg daily (one fourth usual adult dose)

Present D. Duration
1. Less than three days
2. More than two changes of psychotropic medication in any seven-day period

Review If:

Present E. Concomitance
1. Any other antipsychotic drug
2. More than one other psychotropic drug of any class
3. Anticholinergic or antispasmodic GI drugs

Present F. Critical adverse developments
1. Marked sedation or lethargy after one week
2. Urinary retention
3. Syncope
4. Death from any cause
5. Any follow-up laboratory abnormalities during treatment, e.g.
a. Bilirubin level greater than 1.0 mg/dl
b. SGOT level greater than 100 IU/ml
c. WBC count less than 3,000 cu mm
6. Intentional overdose
7. Tardive dyskinesia

Absent G. Critical adjunctive services

Present H. Relative contraindications
1. History of allergy to this drug
2. Myocardial infarction within six weeks
3. History of tardive dyskinesia
4. Age younger than 5 years

Antipsychotic Medications (Nonpsychotic Disorders): Inpatient Criteria

Review If:

Absent A. Common indications (validate by AMA/DHEW criteria if desired)
1. Any neurosis, in a patient with
a. Failure to respond to a benzodiazepine or
b. Undesirable response to a benzodiazepine, or
c. History of abusing sedatives, tranquilizers, or alcohol, or
d. Pronounced suspiciousness, irritability, mood lability, or agitation
2. Psychophysiological disorders
3. Organic brain syndrome without psychosis
4. Mental retardation with severe behavioral disturbance
5. Minimal brain dysfunction (MBD)

Absent B. Minimal documentation (all standard requirements)

Absent C. Dosage range (chlorpromazine equivalents)
1. Patients aged 13 to 65 years: 100 to 400 mg daily
2. Patients aged 65 years or older (except organic brain syndrome): 50 to 200 mg daily (one half usual adult dose)
3. Patients aged 65 years or older (organic brain syndrome): 25 to 200 mg daily
4. Patients aged 5 to 12 years: 25 to 200 mg daily

Present D. Duration
1. Less than three days
2. More than six months
3. More than two changes of psychotropic medication in any seven-day period

Review If:

Present E. Concomitance
1. Any other antipsychotic drug
2. Any benzodiazepine
3. More than one psychotropic drug of any class
4. Anticholinergic or antispasmodic GI medication

Present F. Critical adverse developments
1. No improvement by 60th percentile LOS for diagnosis (or 21st day)
2. Patient still in hospital by 90th percentile LOS for diagnosis (or 28th day)
3. Marked sedation or lethargy after one week
4. Urinary retention
5. Syncope
6. Convulsion
7. Death from any cause
8. Tardive dyskinesia
9. Any follow-up laboratory abnormality
a. Bilirubin level greater than 1.0 mg/dl
b. SGOT level greater than 100 IU/ml
c. WBC count less than 3,000/cu mm

Absent G. Critical adjunctive services
1. Basic laboratory studies on admission
2. ECG on admission for patients older than 65 years of age or with recent history of cardiac disorder

Present H. Relative contraindications
1. History of allergy to this drug
2. History or presence of tradive dyskinesia
3. Age younger than 5 years

Antipsychotic Medications (Nonpsychotic Disorders): Outpatient Criteria

Review If:

Absent A. Common indications (validate by AMA/DHEW criteria if desired)
1. Any neurosis, in a patient with
a. Failure to respond to a benzodiazepine, or
b. Undesirable response to a benzodiazepine, or
c. History of abusing sedatives, tranquilizers, or alcohol, or
d. Pronounced suspiciousness, irritability, or agitation
2. Psychophysiological disorders
3. Organic brain syndrome without psychosis
4. Mental retardation with severe behavior disturbance
5. MBD

Absent B. Minimal documentation (all standard outpatient requirements, plus note every three months about presence or absence of tardive dyskinesia)

Absent C. Dosage range (chlorpromazine equivalents)
1. Patients aged 13 to 64 years: 50 to 400 mg daily
2. Patients aged 65 years or older (except organic brain syndrome): 25 to 200 mg daily (one half usual adult dose)
3. Patients aged 65 years or older (organic brain syndrome): 10 to 100 mg daily (one fourth usual adult dose)
4. Patients aged 5 to 12 years: 10 to 100 mg daily (one fourth usual adult dose)

Present D. Duration
1. Less than three days
2. More than six months
3. More than two changes of psychotropic medication in any seven-day period

Review If:
Present E. Concomitance
1. Any other antipsychotic drug
2. More than one other psychotic drug of any class
3. Anticholinergic or antispasmodic GI medication

Present F. Critical adverse developments
1. Marked sedation or lethargy after one week
2. Urinary retention
3. Syncope
4. Death from any cause
5. Any follow-up laboratory abnormalities during treatment, e.g.
   a. Bilirubin level greater than 1.0 mg/dl
   b. SGOT level greater than 100 IU/ml
   c. WBC count less than 3,000/cu mm
6. Intentional overdose
7. Tardive dyskinesia

Absent G. Critical adjunctive services

Present H. Relative contradindications
1. History of allergy to this drug
2. Myocardial infarction within six weeks
3. History or presence of tardive dyskinesia
4. Age younger than 5 years

Antipsychotic Medications

Generic	Trade Names	Usual Daily Antipsychotic Dosage, mg
1. Chlorpromazine	Chlor-PZ, Cromedazine, Promachel, Thorazine	400-1,600
2. Triflupromazine hydrochloride	Vesprin	100-200
3. Thioridazine	Mellaril	400-800
4. Mesoridazine	Lidanar, Serentil	100-500

5. Piperacetazine	Quide	40-160
6. Acetophenazine maleate	Tindal	60-300
7. Butaperazine	Repoise	20-160
8. Carphenazine maleate	Proketazine	75-400
9. Fluphenazine hydrochloride	Permitil, Prolixin, Trancin	5-40
a. Fluphenazine decanoate	Prolixin Decanoate	12½-100 (every two weeks)
b. Fluphenazine enanthate	Prolixin Enanthate	12½-100
10. Perphenazine	Trilafon	8-64
11. Trifluoperazine Hydrochloride	Stelazine	10-80
12. Chlorprothixene	Taractan	400-1,600
13. Thiothixene	Navane	10-60
14. Haloperidol	Haldol	5-100
15. Molindone hydrochloride	Lidone, Moban	20-225
16. Loxapine succinate	Daxolin, Loxitane	50-250

Fixed-Ratio Combination Products, Amitriptyline-Perphenazine: Inpatient and Outpatient Criteria

Review If:

Absent — A. Common indications (validate by AMA/DHEW criteria if desired)
1. Schizophrenia (any subtype) with
   a. Associated depression, and
   b. Failure to respond to antipsychotic medication alone, and
   c. Prior independent titration of doses of amitriptyline and perphenazine (optional criterion)
2. Manic-depressive illness (depressed type), psychotic depressive reaction, involutional melancholia, or severe depressive neurosis, with
   a. Intense anxiety, agitation, or paranoia, and
   b. Failure to respond to antidepressant medication alone, and
   c. Prior independent titration of doses of amitriptyline and perphenazine (optional criterion)

Absent — B. Minimal documentation (all standard inpatient or outpatient requirements)

Absent — C. Dosage range (Etrafon, Triavil)
1. Age younger than 65 years: 100 to 300 mg daily of amitriptyline component
2. Age older than 65 years: one half the aforementioned dosage

Review If:

Present D. Duration
1. Less than three days
2. More than two changes of psychotropic medication in any seven-day period

Present E. Concomitance
1. Any other psychotropic drug
2. Guanethidine sulfate, clonidine hydrochloride, or bethanidine sulfate

Present F. Critical adverse developments
1. No improvement by 60th percentile LOS for diagnosis
2. Patient still in hospital by 90th percentile LOS for diagnosis
3. Marked sedation or lethargy after one week of treatment
4. Extrapyramidal side effects (acute dystonia, akathesia, pseudoparkinsonian syndrome, tardive dyskinesia)
5. Urinary retention
6. Ileus or persistent constipation
7. Syncope
8. Intentional overdose
9. Death from any cause

Absent G. Critical adjunctive services
1. Basic laboratory studies on admission

Present H. Relative contraindications
1. Known allergies to these drugs
2. Myocardial infarction within six weeks
3. History of acute angle glaucoma
4. History or prescence of tardive dyskinesia
5. Age younger than 12 years

Fixed-Ratio Combination Products, Amitriptyline-Chloradiazepoxide: Inpatient and Outpatient Criteria

Review If:

Absent A. Common indications (validate by AMA/DHEW criteria if desired)
1. Depressive neurosis with
   a. Moderate to severe anxiety and
   b. Prior independent titration of doses of amitriptyline and chlordiazepoxide (optional criterion)

Absent B. Minimal documentation (all standard inpatient or outpatient requirements)

Absent C. Dosage range (Limbitrol)
1. Age younger than 65 years: 100 to 300 mg daily of amitriptyline hydrochloride component
2. Age older than 65 years: 50 to 150 mg daily of amitriptyline hydrochloride component

Present D. Duration
1. Less than three days
2. More than six months
3. More than two changes of psychotropic Medication in any seven-day period

Present E. Concomitance
1. Any other psychotropic drug
2. Guanethidine, clonidine, or bethanidine

Review If:

Present F. Critical adverse developments
1. No improvement by 60th percentile LOS for diagnosis
2. Patient still in hospital by 90th percentile LOS for diagnosis
3. Marked sedation or lethargy after one week of treatment
4. Urinary retention
5. Syncope
6. Ileus or persistent constipation
7. Intentional overdose
8. Death from any cause

Absent G. Critical adjunctive services
1. Basic laboratory studies on admission

Present H. Relative contraindications
1. History of allergy to amitriptyline or chlordiazepoxide
2. Myocardial infarction within six weeks
3. History of acute angle glaucoma
4. Age younger than 12 years

Hypnotic Medications: Inpatient and Outpatient Criteria

Review If:

Absent A. Common indications
1. Insomnia

Absent B. Minimal documentation (all standard inpatient or outpatient requirements)

Absent C. Dosage range
1. Barbiturates
   a. Secobarbital (Seconal), 100 to 200 mg
   b. Pentobarbital (Nembutal), 100 to 200 mg
   c. Butabarbital (Butabarbunicells, Butatab, Butisol, Medarsed), 50 to 200 mg
   d. Amobarbital (Amosed, Amosette, Amytal), 100 to 300 mg
2. Piperidines
   a. Methyprylon (Noludar), 200 to 400 mg
   b. Glutethimide (Doriden), 250 to 1,000 mg
3. Quinazolines
   a. Methaqualone (Parest, Quaalude, Sopor) 150 to 400 mg
4. Acetylinic alcohols
   a. Ethchlorvynol (Placidyl), 500 to 1,000 mg

5. Chloral derivatives
   a. Chloral hydrate (amyiophene, Aquachioral, En-Chlor, Felsules, Kessodrate, Lycoral, Noctec, Rectules, Somnos), 500 to 1,500 mg
6. Benzodiazepines
   a. Flurazepam hydrochloride (Dalmane), 15 to 30 mg

Present D. Duration
1. Seven days continued use

Review If:
Present E. Concomitance
1. With barbiturates and chloral hydrate coumarin anticoagulants, other CNS depressants (e.g. tricyclic antidepressants)
2. More than one other psychotropic medication

Present F. Critical adverse developments
1. Prolonged lethargy
2. Ataxia (especially in elderly)
3. Delirium (confusion and disorientation)
4. Paradoxical excitement
5. Respiratory depression
6. Withdrawal symptoms on discontinuation of therapy
7. Intentional overdose

Absent G. Critical adjunctive services
1. Basic laboratory studies on admission
2. Daily vital signs for inpatients older than 65 years of age

Present H. Relative contraindications
1. History of addiction to sedative or hypnotic drugs
2. With barbiturates: porphyria and impaired hepatic functions
3. With chloral hydrate: marked hepatic and renal impairment
4. Pregnancy (especially first trimester)
5. Known allergy to this group of drugs
6. Age younger than 16 years

Lithium: Inpatient Criteria

Review If:
Absent A. Common indications
1. Manic-depressive illness, manic type
2. Manic-depressive illness, circular type, manic phase
3. Schizoaffective illness, manic type
4. Schizoaffective illness, circular type, manic phase (schizophrenia, schizoaffective type, manic)

Absent B. Minimal documentation (all standard inpatient requirements

Absent C. Dosage range (lithium carbonate)
1. Oral dosage: 600 to 3,600 mg daily
2. Plasma level: 0.6 to 1.5 mEq

Present D. Duration
1. Less than three days
2. More than two changes of psychotropic medication in any seven-day period

Present E. Concomitance
1. More than two other psychotropic drugs of any class
2. Diuretic medication
3. Salt-free diet

Present F. Critical adverse developments
1. No improvement by 60th percentile LOS for diagnosis (or 21st day)
2. Patients still in hospital by 90th percentile LOS for diagnosis (or 28th day)

Review If:
Present
3. Lethargy, stupor, or coma
4. Polyuria and polydipsia
5. Severe tremor lasting seven days
6. Vomiting
7. Nausea or diarrhea for seven or more days
8. Ataxia and dysarthria

Absent F. Critical adjunctive services
1. Daily vital signs
2. Basic laboratory studies on admission, including measure of renal function
3. Serum electrolyte determinations on admission
4. Thyroid function studies on admission
5. Lithium plasma level measurement at least twice in first ten days of treatment

Present H. Relative contraindications
1. History of allergy to this drug
2. Existence of renal failure as reflected by progress note
3. Existence of vomiting as reflected by progress note
4. Existence of dehydration as reflected by progress note
5. BUN level greater than 50 mg/dl
6. Age younger than 12 years
7. Pregnancy or breast-feeding

Lithium: Outpatient Criteria

Review If:
Absent A. Common indications (validate by AMA/DHEW criteria if desired)
1. Manic-depressive illness, manic type
2. Manic-depressive illness, circular type, manic phase
3. Schizoaffective illness, manic type
4. Schizoaffective illness, circular type, manic phase
5. Recurrent manic-depressive illness, circular or manic type, asymptomatic

Absent B. Minimal documentation (all standard outpatient requirements)

Absent C. Dosage range (lithium carbonate)
1. Oral dosage: 600 to 3,600 mg daily
2. Plasma level: 0.6 to 1.5 mEq

Present D. Duration
1. Less than three days
2. More than two changes of psychotropic medication in any seven-day period

Present E. Concomitance
1. With barbiturates and chloral hydrate coumarin anticoagulants, other CNS depressants (e.g. tricyclic antidepressants)
2. More than one other psychotropic medication

Review If:

Present F. Critical adverse developments
1. Lethargy, stupor, or coma
2. Polyuria and polydipsia
3. Severe tremor lasting seven days
4. Vomiting
5. Nausea or diarrhea for seven or more days
6. Ataxia and dysarthria
7. Intentional overdose

Absent G. Critical adjunctive services
1. Laboratory tests for thyroid and renal function and serum electrolyte measurement before initiation of treatment
2. Serum lithium measurement at least twice in the first two weeks of initial treatment
3. Lithium plasma level measurement at least every three months during maintenance therapy

Present H. Relative contraindications
1. History of allergy to this drug
2. Existence of renal failure as reflected by progress note
3. Existence of severe vomiting as reflected by progress note
4. Existence of dehydration as reflected by progress note
5. Age younger than 12 years
6. Pregnancy or breast-feeding

Psychostimulant Medication for Children: Inpatient and Outpatient Criteria

Review If:

Absent A. Indications
1. Minimal brain dysfunction with hyperactivity or distractability
2. Narcolepsy

Absent B. Minimal documentation (all standard inpatient or outpatient requirements)

Absent C. Dosage range
1. Dextroamphetamine (Dexedrine), 5 to 80 mg/day
2. Methylphenidate hydrochloride (Ritalin), 5 to 18 mg/day
3. Penoline Cylert), 37.5 to 150 mg/day

Present D. Duration
1. More than nine months without change in dose

Present E. Concomitance
1. Any other psychostimulant given simultaneously for more than 30 days
2. More than one other psychotropic drug of any class
3. Any MAO inhibitor

Present F. Critical adverse developments
1. No improvement in 30 days
2. Marked sedation or depression
3. Agitation, restlessness, or stimulation
4. Confusion or hallucinations
5. Marked anorexia and weight loss
6. Convulsions
7. Death from any cause

Absent G. Critical adjunctive services
1. Daily vital signs (inpatient only)
2. Basic laboratory studies on admission to hospital
3. Height and weight recordings on initiation of treatment and every three months thereafter
4. Direct contact with child and parent at least every three months

Present H. Relative contraindications
1. Known allergy or adverse response to drug
2. Age younger than 5 years or greater than 18 years

Tricyclic Antidepressants: Inpatient and Outpatient Criteria

Review If:

Absent A. Common indications (validate by AMA/DHEW criteria if desired)
1. Depressive neurosis
2. Manic-depressive illness, depressed type or phase
3. Psychotic depressive reaction
4. Involutional melancholia
5. Pediatric uses
   a. Minimal brain dysfunction
   b. Enuresis
   c. School phobia
   d. Night terrors

Absent B. Minimal documentation (all standard inpatient or outpatient requirements)

Absent — C. Dosage range for adults (half of standard dose if patient is older than 65 years of age)

1. Amitriptyline hydrochloride (Amitril, Domical, Elavil, Endep), 100 to 300 mg/day (ages 5 to 12 years: 25 to 150 mg daily)
2. Desipramine hydrochloride (Norpramin, Pertofrane), 100 to 300 mg/day (ages 5 to 12 years: 25 to 150 mg daily)
3. Doxepin hydrochloride (Adapin, Curatin, Sinequan), 100 to 300 mg/day (ages 5 to 12 years: 25 to 150 mg daily)
4. Imipramine hydrochloride (Imarate, Pramine, Tofranil), 100 to 300 mg/day (ages 5 to 12 years: 25 to 150 mg daily)
5. Nortriptyline (Aventyl Hydrochloride, Pamelor), 50 to 150 mg/day (ages 5 to 12 years: 10 to 75 mg daily)
6. Protriptyline hydrochloride (Triptil, Vivactil), 20 to 60 mg/day (ages 5 to 12 years: 5 to 30 mg daily)

Present — D. Duration

1. Less than three days
2. More than two changes of psychotropic medication in any seven-day period

Review If:

Present — E. Concomitance

1. Any other tricyclic antidepressant
2. MAO inhibitor
3. More than one other psychotropic medication of any class
4. Guanethidine, clonidine, or bethanidine
5. Anticholinergic antiparkinsonian drug
6. Reserpine

Present — F. Critical adverse developments

1. No improvement by local 60th percentile LOS for diagnosis (or 21 days for inpatients, 42 days for outpatients)
2. Patients still in hospital by local 90th percentile LOS for diagnosis (or 28 days)
3. Marked sedation or lethargy after first week
4. Urinary retention
5. Syncope
6. Intentional overdose
7. Psychosis, hallucinosis, or delirium coming on during treatment
8. Death from any cause

Absent — G. Critical adjunctive services

1. Daily vital signs (inpatient only)
2. Basic laboratory studies on admission
3. ECGs on admission for patients older than 65 years of age or with a history of cardiovascular disease

Present — H. Relative contraindications

1. History of allergy to this drug
2. Myocardial infarction within six weeks
3. History of acute angle glaucoma
4. Age younger than 5 years

Monoamine Oxidase Inhibitors: Inpatient and Outpatient Criteria

Review If:

Absent A. Common indications (validate by AMA/DHEW criteria if desired)
1. Depressive neurosis
2. Manic-depressive illness, depressed type or phase
3. Psychotic depressive reaction
4. Involutional melancholia

Absent B. Minimal documentation (all standard inpatient or outpatient requirements)

Absent C. Dosage range
1. Phenelzine sulfate, 30 to 90 mg/day
2. Tranylcypromine sulfate, 30 to 80 mg/day
3. Isocarboxazid, 30 to 80 mg/day

Present D. Duration
1. Less than three days
2. More than two changes of psychotropic medication in any seven-day period

Present E. Concomitance
1. Any other MAO inhibitor
2. Any tricyclic antidepressant
3. Reserpine
4. Any psychostimulant
5. Any drug containing epinephrine or its congeners
6. More than one other psychotropic medication of any class
7. Anticholingergic antiparkinson drug

Review If:

Present F. Critical adverse developments
1. No improvement by loca 60th percentile LOS for diagnosis (or 21 days)
2. Patients still in hospital by local 90th percentile LOS for diagnosis (or 28 days)
3. Marked sedation, lethargy
4. Agitation, restlessness
5. Confusion
6. Severe headache
7. Coma
8. Death from any cause
9. Intentional overdose

Absent G. Critical adjunctive services
1. Basic laboratory studies on admission
2. Vital signs at least once daily
3. ECG for patients older than 40 years of age
4. Tyramine-restricted diet

Present H. Relative contraindications
1. Known allergy to this drug
2. Myocardial infarction within six weeks
3. Age younger than 12 years

Canadian Trade Names of Drugs

Generic Names	Trade Names
Antianxiety Medications	
Chlordiazepoxide hydrochloride	Corax, C-Tran, Dymopoxide, Librium, Medilium, Nack, Novopoxide, Protensin, Relaxil Solium, Trilium
Clorazepate dipotassium	Tranxene
Diazepam	D-Tran, E-Pam, Erital, Meval, Novodipam, Paxel, Neo-Calme, Serenack, Stress-Pam, Valium, Vivol
Lorazepam	Ativan
Meprobamate	Equanil, Lan-Dol, Meditran, Mep-E, Meprospan-400, Miltown, Neo-Tran, Novo-mepro, Probal, Quietal, Trelmar
Oxazepam	Serax
Antiparkinsonism Medications (Except Levodopa)	
Amantadine hydrochloride	Symmetrel
Benztropine mesylate	Cogentin
Biperiden hydrochloride	Akineton
Procyclidine hydrochloride	Kemadrin, Procyclid
Trihexyphenidyl hydrochloride	Aparkane, Artane, Novohexidyl, Trihexy, Trixyl
Antipsychotic Medications	
Chlorpromazine	Chlorprom, Chlor-Promanyl, Chlorprom-Ez-Ets, Largactil
Fluphenazine decanoate	Modecate
Fluphenazine enanthate	Modetin
Haloperidol	Haldol
Loxapine	Loxapac
Mesoridazine besylate	Serentil
Perphenazine	Phenazine, Trilafon
Piperacetazine	Quide
Thioridazine	Mellaril, Novoridazine, Thioril
Thiothixene	Navane
Fixed-Ratio Combination Products	
Amitriptyline-Perphenazine	Etrafon, Triavil
Hypnotic Medications	
Barbiturates	
Amobarbital	Amytal, Sodium Amytal, Isobec
Butabarbital	Butisol, Day-Barb,Neo-Barb
Pentobarbital	Nembutal, Nov-Rectal, Pentogen
Secobarbital	Secogen, Seconal, Seral
Piperidines	
Glutethimide	Doriden
Methyprylon	Noludar

Canadian Trade Names of Drugs (Cont'd.)

Generic Names	Trade Names
Hypnotic Medications Cont'd.	
Quinazolines	
Methaqualone	Hyptor, Mequelon, Methadorm, Quaalude-300, Rouqualone-"300", Sedalone, Triador, Tualone - 300, Vitalone
Acetylinic Alchols	
Ethchlorvynol	Placidyl
Chloral derivatives	
Chloral hydrate	Chloralex, chloralixir, Chloralvan, Noctec, Novochlorhydrate
Benzodiazepines	
Flurazepam hydrochloride	Dalmane
Lithium	
Lithium Carbonate	Carbolith, Lithane, Lithizine
Psychostimulant Medications for Children	
Dextroamphetamine	Dexedrine
Methylphenidate hydrochloride	Methidate, Ritalin
Tricyclic Antidepressants	
Amitriptyline hydrochloride	Amiline, Deprex, Elavil, Levate, Meravil, Novotriptyn
Desipramine hydrochloride	Norpramin, Pertofrane
Doxepin hydrochloride	Sinequan
Imipramine hydrochloride	Impranil, Impril, Novopramine, Praminil, Tofranil
Nortriptyline	Aventyl
Protriptyline hydrochloride	Triptil
Monoamine Oxidase Inhibitors	
Phenelzine Sulfate	Nardil
Tranylcypromine Sulfate	Parnate
Isocarboxazid	Marplan

Discussion of Dorsey's "Peer Review and the Use of Psychotropic Drugs"

A. G. Awad, MB. B. Ch.

Dr. Richard Dorsey is to be congratulated on an elegant and very informative presentation. The use of psychotropic medications is an important issue in the practice of modern psychiatry. The last 25 years have witnessed the introduction of an impressive series of psychopharmacological agents that have dramatically influenced the care and treatment of the psychiatrically ill. Our hospital complex, *Queen Street Mental Health Centre*, is just one witness for that revolution. At the present time our hospital houses less than 400 patients, while only 20 years ago it had over 1500 patients. It is not mere coincidence that the community mental health movement became possible in the early 1950's, the time of the major breakthroughs in psychiatric drug therapy.

Given the extensive use of psychopharmacological agents over the past 25 years, one would expect physicians to have expertise in the proper and rational use of them. Unfortunately, this is not the case. Psychotropic drugs are often prescribed in a way that is not congruent with their pharmacological properties, with the latest research findings, or with the most cost-effective pattern.

Current practices of drug therapy in mental illness have been criticized for being responsible for an unacceptably high level of serious complications such as tardive dyskinesia. On the other hand, the fear instilled in some physicians by such undesirable and dreadful side effects may lead them to undertreat their patients. Denial of treatment because of fear of side effects is a less recognized phenomenon, though all of us will agree that it does take place (1). These are just a few of the many issues encountered in reviewing current practices in drug therapy.

A major factor contributing to this unsatisfactory state of affairs is that most physicians have not received adequate training in psychopharmacology in medical schools. In 1972, a survey of medical schools in the United States revealed that fewer than 20% offered a formal course in clinical psychopharmacology (2). Even psychiatrists, who logically should be better trained and more skilled in the use of psychopharmacological agents, are grossly undertrained (3). In a survey of ten V. A. hospitals in the United States (4), gross deficiencies in prescribing practices were noted:

1) 32% of patients were being given more than one psychotropic drug concomitantly;

2) 10% of patients were receiving dosages in excess of the recommended daily dose;

3) 42% were receiving antiparkinsonian drugs for longer than three months;

4) drug holidays were not utilized to the extent possible.

Closer to home, two years ago Dr. Paul Garfinkel conducted a survey among psychiatric residents in the Department of Psychiatry at the University of Toronto. Nearly half of the psychiatric residents surveyed rated their training in psychopharmacology as only poor to fair (5). I believe that findings like these are suggestive of widespread deficiencies in psychopharmacology training at all levels of medical practice. At the same time, the very few serious studies available have shown that continuing education following the traditional didactic model has disappointingly little effect on physicians' performance.

Because of issues like these, Dr. Dorsey's attempt to develop widely accepted psychopharmacological screening criteria for evaluation is an important and valuable contribution. Though I am aware of the apprehensions, concerns, and limitations of the principle of peer review in general, I believe that the use of psychotropic drugs is particularly accessible to the review process by means of reasonable screening criteria.

One of the frequent criticisms is that evaluative criteria can easily lead to mediocrity in medical practice. From our experience, I do not believe this is the case, provided that everyone understands, as Dr. Dorsey emphasized, that evaluative criteria are not intended to be definitive standards. In our hospital, developing review criteria required intensive discussion, literature review, and review of our current practices. Eventually, this led to cooperation, with many individuals of different theoretical orientations reconciling their differences in favor of a more scientific and rational approach to psychiatric practice. In a presentation to the Canadian Psychiatric Association (6), we reported that those who had participated in the audit process in our hospital rated it as a good educational experience in itself.

This encouraging observation, combined with the identified deficiency in postgraduate training in psychopharmacology, and the inadequacy of traditional teaching models, has led me to experiment with the criteria audit system described by Dr. Dorsey as an educational tool for the training in the proper use of psychopharmacological agents. Modified audits are to be used as a form of teaching seminar in which the residents and their supervisors can participate in the whole process. This should provide useful feedback to the residents about their performance in the use of psychopharmacological agents in a real clinical situation.

I would like to conclude my remarks on Dr. Dorsey's excellent presentation by quoting from a recent article in Lancet by the Professor of Surgery at Cambridge University (7)

> it is anomalous that the day a man ceases to be a senior registrar on his appointment as a consultant marks the beginning of a period, extending to retirement age, in which professional criticism from his colleagues is most unlikely, unless his malpractice is so blatant as to involve a suit for damage.......First-class and very bad surgeons tend to be known by their colleagues, particularly their junior staff. Yet a surgeon may spend his whole life making poor judgements and operating badly with an unacceptably high morbidity and mortality, and remain unaware that his work is below par.

Surely these remarks about surgeons apply to psychiatrists and other medical specialists as well.

REFERENCES

1. Shader, R.I., Fear of side effects and denial of treatment; Rational psychopharmacotherapy and the right to treatment, 106-117, ed. F. J. Ayd, Ayd Medical Communications, (1975).

2. DiMascio A., Innovative drug administration regimens and the economics of mental health care; Rational psychopharmacotherapy and the right to treatment, 118-130, ed. F. J. Ayd, Ayd Medical Communications, (1975).

3. Gottlieb, R. M., Nappi, T., and Strain, J. J., The physician's knowledge of psychotropic drugs: Preliminary results. Am. J. Psychiatry, 135: 29-32, (1978).

4. GAO Report to the Congress, Controls needed to help assure appropriate use of drugs used to treat psychiatric patients, and improvements needed in Psychiatrist Staffing. Washington, D. C.: U. S. Government Printing Office, (1970).

5. Garfinkel, P. E., Cameron, P., Kingstone, E., Psychopharmacology education in psychiatry, Can. J. Psychiatry, 24: 644-651, (1979).

6. Awad, A. G., Durost, H. B., Gray, J., Kugelmass, M., Smith, C., Psychiatric Audits - The Ontario Scene, Can. J. Psychiatry: in press.

7. Calne, R., Surgical self-scrutiny, Lancet ii, 1309, (1974).

Peer Review of Outpatient Psychological Services

George Stricker, Ph.D.

The traditional arena for the peer review of mental health services has been the hospital. Where review has been other than local in scope, it has fallen under the auspices of Professional Standards Review Organizations (PSRO), and has dealt exclusively with the care received by federal patients in inpatient facilities (1). To date, most review systems have focussed on matters such as criteria for admission and continued stay review.

I would like to describe a practical application, national in scope, of quality assurance principles in an ambulatory care setting. This project has been undertaken by the American Psychological Association under contract from the Civilian Health and Medical Program for the Uniform Services (CHAMPUS). CHAMPUS is a health plan with over seven million beneficiaries. It covers retired military personnel, dependents of active duty military personnel and, in some instances, active duty servicemen. The mental health budget of CHAMPUS is over 100 million dollars, representing close to 20% of the entire budget of the program. Of this mental health budget, almost 20% is concerned with outpatient care (2). The plan provides an appropriate model for third party payers: the co-payment is small, there is no benefit ceiling, and the only criterion for continued coverage is that the service be either medically or psychologically necessary.

---

* Members of the National Advisory Panel include George Stricker, Chair, Russell Bent, Vice-Chair, Anna Rosenberg, Lee Sechrest, Joan Willens, Harl Young and William Claiborn, Project Director. Melvin Gravitz initially served on the Panel and resigned after the first year.

CHAMPUS began covering mental health services in 1966, accepting psychologists as independent providers along with physicians. After several years of experience with mental health coverage, a public furor arose concerning care in residential treatment centres. It was clear that substandard facilities, often staffed by untrained and inadequate people, were drawing federal funds to "treat" needy patients. In response to this problem, CHAMPUS established a Select Committee on Psychiatric Care Evaluation (SCOPCE I), an interdisciplinary body charged with setting standards of care for residential treatment centres. The document that it produced resulted in the withdrawal of funds from almost 90% of the facilities that had been providing services. This dramatic effect of professionally established criteria meant great cost savings but, more importantly, it significantly raised the quality of service available to the beneficiaries. Since substandard facilities had been eliminated, the patients who sought care were assured of the quality of their treatment.

Because of the SCOPCE experience, CHAMPUS was receptive to establishing professional criteria for peer review of services. In the mid-1970's CHAMPUS raised a question in the Congress about the continued funding of mental health services and the inadequacy of existing review mechanisms. Accordingly, CHAMPUS agreed to establish National Advisory Panels, and in July, 1977 signed contracts with the American Psychological Association to establish criteria for the review of outpatient mental health services (3). This action was similar to the SCOPCE model in that the professional community was to establish standards to guide review decisions, but it differed in that two committees were formed, one from each independent provider profession as CHAMPUS preferred to avoid the issue of healing the rifts between psychiatry and psychology. An alternative to this fairly enlightened approach, which other insurance companies and National Health Insurance might take, is to tell the professions that if they cannot work together, they will not be allowed to work separately. I would much prefer to see an effort made in common, in an interdisciplinary fashion. To the extent that this is not done, each profession may be risking its future with third party payers.

The problem that faced CHAMPUS is shared by third party payers. In a classic book on the theory of psychoanalytic technique, Menninger and Holzman (4) present treatment almost entirely from the point of view that psychotherapy is a two-party contract. They examine the obligations and expectations of both parties, consider how distortions in these can affect the treatment process, and describe how one can learn about characteristic modes of functioning from these distortions. This philosophy--that psychotherapy is a two-party contract, and that whatever occurs in the consultation room is confidential between the patient and the therapist--is shared by a great many therapists regardless of discipline. Now, however, a third party has entered the system. Over half of the psychotherapy currently being conducted in the United States is being funded by a party other than the patient or the patient's immediate family (5). Mental health professionals as a group have welcomed the entrance of the third party, because services have become accessible to a much broader segment of the population. These same professionals, however, have been loathe to share with that party any information about the nature of the services that are being performed, for that would disrupt the confidentiality of the therapist-patient relationship.

This approach can only be tenable if insurance companies are philanthropic associations. To the extent that they are not, they will find the situation increasingly intolerable as the budget mounts. Decisions about the payment of claims must be made. They can be made by the third party payer on the basis of actuarial criteria, which will lead to large co-payments and clear restrictions on services. Alternatively, the decisions can be made by professionals on a clinical basis. The third party payer currently controls decisions about the beneficiaries and the authorization of providers. The crucial question facing us was how to determine which services are appropriate; we have proceeded on the assumption that such decisions should be made by professionals, on the basis of clinical criteria.

CHAMPUS regulations placed a number of constraints on psychology's National Advisory Panel. For example, there are retrospective, concurrent, and prospective review systems. The panel favored prospective review: studying a service plan, authorizing the service in advance, and then allowing both the patient and the provider to continue on the understanding that the service would be reimbursable. CHAMPUS regulations, however, require that review be retrospective: reviewing services that have already been offered. Regulations also established the review points: review must occur at the 8th, 24th, 40th, and 60th sessions. In addition, peer review is required whenever a case reaches 60 sessions, or whenever a patient is seen more than twice a week.

Within this structure, the Panel opted for a system which would review exceptions, as this was the only manageable approach. The number of claims filed each year is so large that there is no conceivable way that each case could be reviewed, even if we had wished it. Instead, we established a system in which information would be filed at mandated review points and examined by reviewers in the utilization review office of the fiscal intermediary. As in the PSRO model these reviewers, frequently nurses, would then decide whether or not cases should be sent on to a psychologist peer reviewer, basing their decisions on the explicit criteria that we had constructed.

When a case is pulled out for review, all the identifying information on the patient and the provider is removed, and the case is sent to three reviewers who make their decisions independently. The choice of three reviewers, again, is a contractual constraint placed upon us. I suspect that a sequential review strategy would be better, accepting a positive decision by a single reviewer, and using additional reviewers only in the event of a denial. The Panel is currently researching the process of review decisions, and we expect to make an empirically based recommendation on the appropriate number of reviewers. In any case, the peer reviewers are not given explicit criteria, but are asked to use their best professional judgement in arriving at decisions about the quality and appropriateness of service. Eventually, also on the basis of research, the clinical literature, and the history of review decisions, we hope to establish guidelines for our professional peer reviewers. Thus, we would like to move from implicit to explicit criteria wherever possible.

Several principles guided our decisions in setting up a review system. First, the review system should be helpful to the beneficiary, the provider, and CHAMPUS, and flexible enough to change as we received feedback about its operation. Secondly, the system should concentrate on the goals of treatment and follow progress toward these goals by successive evaluations, using clear behavioral and descriptive terms. Thus, the expected and the actual outcomes of service could be compared, and progress followed. Thirdly, while the system would allow for a wide range of treatment orientations, we should try to develop standard definitions and criteria for treatment planning, intervention methods, and evaluation of care which would apply to all orientations. Fourthly, the patient should be involved both in setting goals and evaluating results; this would lead to a more specific contract of understanding between the patient and the psychologist. Finally, psychiatric diagnosis should not serve as the basis for the psychology system of peer review. This may be the most progressive and the most controversial aspect of our system; certainly it is a major point of divergence from the approach of our psychiatric colleagues. These last two important principles--the active involvement of the patient in treatment planning and evaluation, and the lack of reliance on traditional diagnostic nomenclature--will be treated in greater detail as the system is outlined.

It is important to emphasize that our criteria are designed for utilization reviewers, and that they represent our estimate of usual and customary practice (6, 7). We have not attempted to write regulations; we have selected exceptions which appear to be in need of professional scrutiny. It is entirely possible that services outside our criteria will be reimbursed if a panel of peers can be convinced that even though a service was not customary, given the clinical nature of the case it was appropriate.

At each of the mandated review points the therapist is asked to fill out a treatment report, which includes a description of the problem, a statement of goals, a statement of proposed interventions, and an account of progress since the last review point. We do not ask for detailed historical material, for elaborate psychodynamic formulations, or for detailed progress notes, but we do expect sufficient information, stated in explicit behavioral terms, to allow a utilization reviewer, and perhaps eventually a peer reviewer, to arrive at a decision about the quality and the appropriateness of the care rendered. The burden for providing the information is on the provider; if information is absent, reviewers are instructed to assume that that information does not exist. Thus, if their cases are denied because of insufficient documentation, providers will quickly learn what information is needed.

The problem must be stated in sufficient detail so that the reviewers can determine whether the treatment was necessary. It should describe the circumstances, frequency, degree of disruption, and point of onset of the problem. It must include evidence of either significant functional impairment or significant personal distress, making it clear that the patient is unable to function effectively in at least one of the following areas: home or family, job or school, personal relationships, bodily function, protection of self and/or others, and personal comfort. This emphasis on impairment stems from CHAMPUS regulations, which require that in order to qualify for reimbursement, mental health services be restorative rather than for personal growth. This restriction should make it clear that services not included in the criteria may still be professionally appropriate.

Since the statement of the problem is a substitute for diagnosis, and defines the necessity for service, it is important that it be stated clearly and in behavioral terms. A presenting problem such as "depression" would not be sufficient, whereas a statement such as "the patient feels continuing sadness associated with the loss of role clarity due to the growing independence of children" would make the need for services far more clear.

Similarly, a goal such as "the patient will feel better" would not allow for informed review, while a statement such as "the patient will have reported substantial relief from personal distress, including feeling calmer, less tense, better able to handle stress, and eating and sleeping regularly" could easily be used as a criterion for progress. This last example illustrates the need for goals to be stated in concrete terms, to be clearly related to the presenting problem, and to be stated in terms of change expected by the next review point. The goals also must be reasonably attainable through psychotherapeutic processes.

There are very clear reasons as to why we did not incorporate diagnosis into the system. For a diagnostic system to be of value, it must be used by practitioners as a reliable means of determining treatment programs. Although research indicates that if used by appropriately trained professionals, diagnostic nomenclature can be a great deal more reliable than most people assume (8), in practice this is rarely the case. Experience with outpatient mental health services shows that four diagnostic categories (anxiety, depression, situation reaction, and behavior disorder) account for almost 90% of the claims that are received. The therapist often makes a conscious decision to circumvent the system and to protect the patient by submitting the most benign diagnosis conceivable. Given the nature of insurance review, in some cases this is an understandable decision, since the claims forms go through the personnel office in the patient's place of employment. However, using an inappropriate label as an entry point to review is an approach that is doomed to failure.

Whatever the motivation for assigning a diagnosis, and even if the claim does not go through the personnel office, as is the case with CHAMPUS, there still is considerable doubt as to whether different diagnoses indicate different courses of treatment. If we examine the PSRO criteria (9), which are diagnosis based, it immediately becomes apparent that each one of the criteria sets for the various diagnoses are virtually identical. The criteria do not indicate a single significant distinction between treatments except for medication. For psychotherapy as well, the same rules apply regardless of diagnosis. Even though there is general insistence on using diagnosis as the point of entry for review, diagnosis is not a differential basis for treatment expectations.

Second to the absence of diagnosis, perhaps the most innovative aspect of our criteria, and another area in which our approach differs radically from the psychiatric approach, is patient participation. The treatment report form requires an estimate of progress by the patient, and the patient's signature, to indicate that the treatment report has been read and accepted. Thus, the patient will be a clear party to a therapeutic contract, and will be aware of the types of services offered and the goals of those services. Occasionally clinical considerations contraindicate such signature, and for those instances, the therapist will attach an explanatory note. However, in the great majority of cases we expect to receive the patient's endorsement of the plan. If we find, through profile analysis, that some therapists state that it would be therapeutically contraindicated for every single one of their patients to sign, that would clearly be a cause for review.

Some limitations upon service are based on CHAMPUS regulations rather than on Panel judgements as to clinical efficacy. Interventions such as sex therapy or training analysis, for example, fall outside of the regulations and would not be reimbursable. Whatever interventions are indicated must be related to the goals and problems stated elsewhere in the treatment report.

There are a number of time limitations, some contained in the regulations and others devised by the Panel. Individual therapy sessions must have a duration of 60 minutes or less, must total two hours a week or less, and must occur at least once every two months. Marital and family sessions must be between 45 and 90 minutes. Group therapy must occur in a group of four to ten enrolled members, with patients eight years of age or older, and must last 60 to 120 minutes. In order to treat a child, the patient must be at least four years of age, and the treatment plan must show collateral involvement with a significant person in the patient's life.

Some of the above limitations can be waived in a therapeutic emergency. An emergency is an abrupt and substantial change in behavior, usually associated with a clear precipitating situation, and involves severe impairment of functioning or marked increase in personal distress. During such a clinical emergency the frequency and duration of treatment may be increased, but there is a limit of eight emergency sessions within each episode of care.

The peer reviewers might also waive the limitations in other circumstances if the psychologist can present explicit and appropriate clinical reasons for deviation. Thus, the review system is a basic framework for customary treatment, which allows appropriate deviations to be approved by peers.

One set of criteria with a great potential for limiting abuse covers multiple treatment for members of the same family. A single provider may not treat more than one member of the same family in an individual psychotherapy session, although there is no limit on joint treatment such as family or marital psychotherapy. One reason for this criterion is clinical, and relates to the desirability of establishing a relationship with a single patient, uncomplicated by obligations to related individuals. This criterion, however, was also established in order to halt abuses that were cited to the Panel. There have been reports of single providers seeing a number of members of the same family many times during a week, so that a single family might receive dozens of hours of service from one provider in any given week. A reduction in this practice will control costs, and it should also increase the quality of service offered to the patient, since this pattern does not usually appear to be sound practice.

Although we expect that implementation of our review system will result in some cost savings, our goal was not to save money, but rather to improve the quality of service. Quality and cost containment are the twin goals of accountability, they need not be polarized, and hopefully, any decision made on the basis of one approach may also promote the other.

As of this writing (August 1979), CHAMPUS has not implemented our review system, but will most likely begin using it in the fall. The Aetna Insurance Company, however, implemented parts of the system on July 1, 1979. Thus, our work provided a model for health insurance in the private sector even though it was prepared for the public sector.

A national review system has very clear and important implications, some for the provider, some for the patient, and some for the profession. For the _provider_ it will mean filling out a treatment report form at specified intervals. It will require more detailed record-keeping than most private practitioners currently do, although it probably will still fall short of what they ought to do and what most state codes of professional conduct mandate they must do.

Because information will be sent to a third party, the review procedures had to address the question of confidentiality. Occasionally, when practitioners state that they cannot give information because it is confidential, they may mean that they do not want to give the information because they do not want anyone to know what they are doing, or to tell them what to do. In fact, if one were interested in obtaining material about patients, there are richer sources of data than a document filed with an insurance company, such as direct subpoena of the provider. In any case, a number of protections for confidentiality have been built into the system. Documents are kept in separate files, may not be copied or microfilmed except for review purposes, are only distributed with all names deleted, and are destroyed when the treatment episode and period for appeal of claims decisions has expired. In addition, since our system requires the great majority of patients to sign the treatment report form, the patient knows what was said about him, and approves it being released.

The criteria do not define what services are appropriate, but merely what services are reimbursable, the implementation of this system may lead to some restrictions on paid services. Most professionals would agree that a stage in treatment arises with patients where the rehabilitation has essentially been accomplished but the patient continues in treatment for personal growth. Since the CHAMPUS benefit is restorative, and not for growth, claims for such continued service would be disallowed. It should be emphasized that we would not suggest to the professional that the practice is inappropriate, but rather that the patient should understand that treatment has entered a new stage. I do expect, however, that alterations in benefits will affect patterns of practice; therapists will probably practice more of what is reimbursable by a third party, and less of what is reimbursable by the patient whose resources are far more limited.

The effects of the review system on the _patient_ are considerable. The system goes beyond Menninger's "implicit contract," and for the first time makes the patient a party to an explicit contract with the therapist. In addition, there should be higher quality of service available to the patient as substandard services are dropped, as was true in the case of the residential treatment centres. Whereas patients have traditionally relied on the integrity of their provider for the services that they received, there will now be external comment on those services. Most providers offer treatment with a high degree of integrity, but not always with skills to match. There now will be an external source that will inform the provider, and therefore the patient, whenever the service falls below professionally acceptable levels.

The implications for the profession include the development of clear criteria for practice and probably modifications in training, because it is unlikely that institutions will continue to train students in services that will not be reimbursable or are not considered by the profession to be of high quality. I also expect that the review system will expand to other health plans. If the Aetna experiment works, a number of other insurance plans probably will adopt the same approach. National Health Insurance, if it should occur, and if it should include a mental health benefit, almost certainly will use some system of accountability. If there is an effective system in place, it stands to reason that it will be adopted.

Aside from the practical and professional implications of our work, we are proud that we have helped psychology to take a major step toward public responsibility. We have accepted the burden of accountability in a way that will be in the best interest of our patients. This explicit accountability, which is built into our system, is a source of pride to all of us who have helped to develop this exciting approach to the peer review of mental health services.

REFERENCES

1. Goran, M. J., Roberts, J. S., Kellogg, M. A., Fielding, J. and Jessee, W., The PSRO hospital review system. Medical Care, 13 suppl., (1975).

2. Dörken, H., CHAMPUS ten-state claim experience for mental disorder: Fiscal year 1975. American Psychologist, 32, 697, (1977).

3. Claiborn, W. L. and Stricker, G., PSROs, peer review, and CHAMPUS, Professional Psychology, (in press).

4. Menninger, K. A. and Holzman, P.S., Theory of Psychoanalytic Technique, (2nd ed.), Basic Books, New York, (1973).

5. Dörken, H. and Webb, J. P., Health service practice of licensed/certified psychologists: Training, mobility, clientele, fee-for service practice and hospital practice; Paper presented at the Southeastern Psychological Association, Atlanta, (1978).

6. Stricker, G., Personality assessment and insurance reimbursement, Journal of Personality Assessment, 42, 317, (1978).

7. Stricker, G., Criteria for insurance review of psychological services, Professional Psychology, 10, 118 (1979).

8. Matarazzo, J. D., The interview: Its reliability and validity in psychiatric diagnosis. In B. B. Wolman (ed.) Clinical diagnosis of mental disorders: A handbook, Plenum, New York, (1978).

9. PSRO Program Manual, DHEW office of professional standards review, Rockville, Maryland, (1974).

Discussion of Stricker's "Peer Review of Outpatient Psychological Services"

Barry Willer, Ph.D.

There has been a tendency to view quality assurance as a panacea. It has also been presented as a value-free, objective approach to evaluation of the quality of health services. The fact is, however, that no evaluative approach is value-free, and quality assurance is no exception. In fact, quality assurance is in the middle of conflict between competing models of health care delivery. Dr. Stricker's description of the development of quality assurance standards by a subcommittee of the American Psychological Association represents an attempt to develop fair and reasonable standards for outpatient mental health services. It also represents a further conflicting model for mental health service delivery. This paper will attempt to clarify the conflict among models and also point out the implicit values they represent.

Quality assurance was developed in the United States because of the rapidly rising costs of health care. Its primary focus was cost containment, but it has been couched in more palatable terms of quality because the United States lacks the organizational structure and relatively closed-ended financing characteristic of health insurance or health service systems in European countries and Canada.

Anderson says that quality assurance is essentially a compromise between conflicting forces (1). On one side are the insurance companies, politicians, and bureaucrats, who want to put a lid on rapidly rising costs while retaining the rights of all persons to receive quality care. On the other side is the medical profession, which wants to retain control of health services with relatively little interference from government or third party payers. Quality assurance is a compromise in that the *procedures* for evaluation have been developed by those concerned with rising costs, while the *criteria* for evaluation have been developed by professionals and review is conducted by fellow physicians.

The concern for cost containment meant that initial quality assurance procedures and criteria were developed for inpatient services. Only recently has there been discussion of quality assurance procedures for outpatient services since these are generally much less costly. However, with the current movement to develop quality assurance standards for outpatient mental health services, a third interest group has become involved: the non-physicians. Even a cursory examination of the review standards presented by Stricker reveals a vast departure from the language and standards of review developed by physicians. Instead of diagnosis, prognosis, and symptoms, Stricker talks of needs, goals, and outcomes. In fact, Stricker and the American Psychological Association committee have carefully omitted any discussion of diagnosis, which is the basis for all decision making in the medical model.

Conflicting Models of Mental Health Care

An excellent discussion of the conflicting models of Mental Health care is presented by DuMas (2). He describes three models presently competing for power within the mental health delivery system of the United States. The most familiar is the medical model, which places primary importance on the physician/patient relationship. Until recently, "health care has been a physician-dominated enterprise, in which the medical treatment of disease under a private, fee-for-service system has been emphasized" (3). The non-medical model assumes that persons needing mental health services are not mentally ill(and therefore cannot be diagnosed), but are adapting to their environment in a manner which conflicts with society's norms. The non-medical model assumes that mental health services can be provided by a range of professionals, while the medical model assumes that treatment can only be administered by a physician. These are only two of the major differences between the medical model and the non-medical model which have significance for standards and review procedures in quality assurance.

The third competing model of health care is the antimedical model. DuMas (2) suggests that the antimedical model has developed because of the rapidly rising costs of health care and because health care itself has become a major business activity. The antimedical model represents a shift from the professions to administration: control of health care services will rest in the hands of administrators rather than mental health professionals. In the antimedical model providers of service are expected to have a minimum of training and expertise, and control of quality (cost containment) will be based on (bureaucratic)review rather than professional ethics.

All three models can be found among quality assurance procedures. The procedures for review and review itself grew out of the antimedical model. Criteria for inpatient services were established by physicians in keeping with the medical model. Criteria for outpatient mental health services, for example Stricker's criteria, were based on the non-medical model.

DuMas warns that the antimedical model may become the operational model of the future. Although he does not discuss quality assurance directly, he would probably agree that quality assurance is a major step in that direction. If physicians and other professionals retain and exercise the right to establish criteria for review, they remain in a position to sabotage the entire procedure (1). However, this will only slow the process down--it will in no way end the involvement of political and bureaucratic bodies in the delivery of health services.

Quality Assurance from a Canadian Perspective

The purpose of this symposium is to examine the procedures of quality assurance, and presumably there is some thought being given to the applicability of quality assurance to mental health care in Canada. The purpose of this paper has been to comment on the values inherent in quality assurance. If quality assurance procedures are to be developed in Canada, the persons responsible for establishing the standards must be cognizant of the values being imposed.

As pointed out earlier, quality assurance is an American phenomenon. It was developed in the United States to solve some problems in the health care delivery system that are not unique to the United States, but are certainly different in scope. The standards and procedures have also developed in a manner consistent with the values and models most prevalent in the United States. The question is: Do we need to import quality assurance procedures to Canada and, if so, in what form?

There are major differences between Canada and the United States in the way in which health care is delivered. For example, Stricker points out that half of the psychotherapy services in the United States are funded by third party payers. Government sponsored health care insurance in Canada funds a much larger percentage of mental health services. In Canada, the belief that health care is a right, not a privilege, is in direct contrast to the prevalent attitude in the United States. The medical model, as DuMas (2) describes it, is still in vogue in Canada, and has not been as eroded by proponents of the non-medical and antimedical models. Physicians in medical schools are taught to be personally responsible for the quality of care, while physicians in the United States are taught to be entrepreneurial technicians.

In short, Canada's health care system is very different from that of the United States. The differences are not always readily apparent because of the similarities in language, but they do exist. Canadians must cautiously consider new approaches to system monitoring, such as quality assurance. They should re-examine the original intent of quality assurance, and decide which procedures will best meet their needs. And they must ensure that the procedures are consistent with the values of Canadians and Canadian health professionals.

The purpose of quality assurance is twofold. First and foremost is cost containment. Second is quality control. Canada's health care costs have been rising as rapidly as in the United States, and therefore some procedures for cost containment are necessary. The need for quality control is less easily measured. If we cannot define the need, how can we establish the criteria for necessary services and care of high quality? The issue of quality may, in fact, be better discussed separately from the issue of cost containment.

Quality assurance procedures such as utilization review are, indeed, good procedures for cost containment. They are not the only procedures, however. For example, one could imagine a cost containment procedure that would allow much greater participation by consumers (3). Currently, consumers are not participants in the review procedures, although they are supposed to be represented to some extent by the third-party payers. Another approach to cost containment might concentrate on system changes, such as more government involvement in the supply and demand of health services. Government attempts to close hospitals or change the types of services provided by hospitals have not been popular, but these are probably the most efficient ways to reduce cost. The point is, if the problem is cost containment, various approaches should be considered; there is no need to blindly accept quality assurance procedures.

The second purpose for quality assurance, improving the quality of care, can also be viewed from other perspectives. Before considering ways to assure quality, we need to be sure quality is a problem. What are the indicators of poor quality? As it is currently practiced, quality assurance places a great deal of emphasis on medical records and the development of standards to judge the quality of care from records. At times, the original purpose of quality care has been replaced by the desire for the records to reflect the values of those who developed the standards. Stricker's standards for outpatient services are likely to be highly acceptable to psychologists but are not likely to be acceptable to physicians.

This discussion of Stricker's presentation may seem to be cynical, but it is intended only to be cautionary. Quality assurance is not a value-free operation. The introduction of quality assurance requirements in the United States is part of the general movement toward the antimedical model. Perhaps there are certain aspects of quality assurance procedures now being employed in the United States which can be modified to suit Canadian values. Perhaps there are other more efficient means to attain the same ends.

REFERENCES

1. Anderson, O. W., PSROs, the medical profession, and the public interest. Health and Safety, 379-388, (1976).

2. DuMas, F. M., Medical, non-medical or antimedical models for mental health centres? American J. Psychiatry, 131, 875-878, (1974).

3. Pecarchik, R., Ricci, E., and Nelson, B., Potential contribution of consumers to an integrated health care system, Public Health Reports, 91, 72-76, (1976).

Panel and General Discussion

Tape Transcript

Moderator: Dr. F. H. Lowy

Dr. John Hoenig (St. John's, Nfld.) It is obvious from these presentations this morning that the professions are going in for a major industry which will require, and has already absorbed, an enormous amount of manpower, time--one wonders sometimes how much time is left to speak to patients--and also an enormous amount of cost. Now, people who foster this kind of activity, who put their hearts and souls into it, are evaluators. I would like to ask the panel whether there are any good studies which have shown that a hospital that practices evaluation of peer review is providing better services to their patients. Or is there any study, good or bad, which tries to find out whether it makes any difference whatsoever?

Dr. Stricker. On the contrary--unfortunately, I know of work that says the opposite. Most of the work that has been done so far seems to indicate that evaluation just isn't worth the effort. Hopefully, we can attribute this to the state of the art, and things will get better. Whether they will or not, I don't know of any evidence to supply you with in response to your question.

Dr. Fifer. I hate to keep quoting Brook (1, 2, 3) all day. It sounds as though he is the only person who has ever written a word in the quality assurance literature, but he said evaluation is a 250 million dollar a year business, which is a big business. But then we have lots of children who are graduating from college now or are otherwise unemployed, and evaluation is a new field. That's how we create work. The Joint Commission has been seriously taken to task because they implemented this system coast to coast in seven thousand of our hospitals--while five thousand they accredited--and they didn't really do a pilot first to find out if this increased the quality of care. Many people now say, "Gee, they should have at least made an effort". But, it wasn't made. I would agree with Dr. Stricker--I know of no literature that says that a hospital that audits together, stays together.

Dr. Sibley. I think that's the key question frankly, and I think it does partly represent the state of the art. We get very confused when we start talking about quality of care and quality assessment. We tend to throw those words around more loosely than we should. If we are really looking at it in a fairly rigorous way, it's very difficult to demonstrate that audit makes a difference in patient outcome in some measurable way. There are many audit studies which show that audits improve behavior of the physician. Taking blood pressure twice a day instead of every second day may not change the outcome of patient's hypertension,but it can score well on audit. Now that's an extreme statement. I think it's a little bit like mandating that we should cure cancer when we don't have the strategies yet and we're not quite sure about the size of the problem. Yet that is not sufficient reason to stand back and say we're not going to do anything about cancer. I think there is a really urgent issue to address in evaluation of care, and it requires a great deal of research and study. I don't think we can stand back and do nothing. If we do, I think we'll find ourselves in a situation where the legislative arm of the public or some imaginative bureaucrat will simply state, under the guise of utilization studies, that thou shalt do this and that, and assume that those activities will have some bearing on quality of care. That's the big danger if we don't accept our public accountability.

Dr. Dorsey. I think it's worth putting quality assurance and medicine in perspective. You can talk about all the time and effort going into it, and yet if you compare that with the accounting profession for business, we're not putting as much time and effort into auditing ourselves as General Motors or the Government of Canada--in just keeping tract of their money in proportion to what they're doing. I think that across the Board, what auditing can do in medicine, and probably what it can do in most areas, is to make it much more difficult to do very bad things. It doesn't make it impossible. There are great scandals in business and government notwithstanding long established audit techniques, but it's much more difficult. I think in medicine it takes time and effort but it's possible to constrain very bad practitioners. We're doing this with our own PSRO's in the United States, ultimately disqualifying them from receiving any money out of federal programs, which is an effective sanction. I think it's also helpful to try to look at medicine from the perspective of the public, just as many of us look at the airline industry. The United States has taken a view, for example, that it's worth grounding all of our DC-10 airliners just on the chance that a second one will be defective and crash and kill another 270 some people. So I'm saying that in medicine, too, the public wants not only demonstrated efficacy, but wants people to have done everything possible, whether it works or not, in order to give them the best chance for protecting themselves and not having their lives put at risk.

Dr. Durost. I just want to mention something that I omitted in my hurried passage through my paper this morning. Dr. Fifer reminded me of it a moment ago in his last diagram. There's a recently published manual called "Consolidated Standards for Child, Adolescent, and Adult Psychiatric, Alcoholism, and Drug Abuse Program" that has a section in it--Section 11--called "Quality Assurance". It has six components of quality assurance: evaluation, evaluation and clinical privileges, professional growth and development activities, utilization reviews, individual case reviews, and patient care audit. As Dr. Fifer said, this is a circular feedback process--in each of the first five the standards keep reminding the people who are attempting to apply them that none of them are meaningful unless what action is taken is related directly to the problems identified in the sixth. And I suppose another comment that might be worthwhile--again, it's chauvinistic--is that Canadians have been watching what's been going on below the border, and the PSRO's in Texas are good learning experiences for us. The Canadian Council has been moving quite slowly, but I suspect that that's probably not an inappropriate thing to do, given what we've been hearing this afternoon.

Dr. Stricker. One more methodological note on that: one possibility is that a review mechanism will be self-correcting, so that you won't see a lot of changes. In the early New Mexico experience, one thing they found was that in the first crack, say the first six months, there was a reduction in a number of inappropriate activities; they just immediately dropped out. From then on, there were no changes. But one wonders if there wasn't such a mechanism in effect, if the same behaviors would have dropped out. So the idea that someone is watching may help.

Dr. Dorsey. To take that one step further: in fact PSRO's have "focussed out", which means stopped reviewing. As a result, some of the things that had dropped out dropped back in. So I'm saying again that part of the whole point of auditing in business or in medicine or airlines or whatever is not simply to catch bad things but to try to keep bad things from happening in the first place.

Dr. Fifer. May I say something about that Hawthorne effect? That's very, very important. When we say nothing has happened in the U.S., that's not right. The pattern of medical practice has changed dramatically. We can't document the 'post hoc ergo proptor hoc' argument, but you can't get a tonsillectomy in the United States anymore, and ten years ago you could get your tonsils whipped out readily. Right now uteri are apparently raining from our skies... My prediction is that you're going to have a lot of difficulty getting a hysterectomy in ten years. There are immense shifts in medical care behaviors going on, and while many of them are not directly attributable to an audit, the process--the involvement of the whole medical profession in something called self-evaluation--has a whole lot of spin-offs. We can't directly take credit for them, but boy, there's a lot of change going on in the ways physicians deal with patients now.

you might say that a lot of that is discretionary, but it's certainly a move in the direction of major changes in the incidence, the rates of surgical procedures, that cannot be explained by anything more than just the existence of the surveillance apparatus in many dimensions. It's really important to keep this in mind.

Dr. Lowy. There is one thing I'd better do for the audience. Several people, particularly Dr. Fifer and Dr. Durost, have mentioned the work of Dr. Brook in this field. His work is perhaps not familiar to everybody here, and I can give you two references if anyone is interested. He is R. H. Brook, and (1) is in the New England Journal of Medicine, Vol. 288, p. 1323, 1973. More recently Brook wrote a chapter in a book (2). The book is called Roads to Assurance in Medical Care, edited by Gordon McLachlan, Oxford University Press, 1976, and the chapter is entitled "Quality Assurance Mechanisms in the United States, from There to Where?"

Dr. Sibley. There is a third reference which is very appropriate to what we are doing here. I think it was in the Annals of Internal Medicine in 1976,(3) in which he looked at the present state of quality assurance research, and brought in eight recommendations for future research activities, trying to lay down a plan for the next eight to ten years. It's very provocative and bears very much on some of the issues we're talking about here now.

Dr. McCormick (Toronto). My question is directed most obviously to Dr. Dorsey, but I suppose there are parallels in other fields. I want to know how you draw the line in what you wouldn't approve of as experts but you find as common practice. Now, I can quite see that you wrote up criteria for the combination of trycyclic and neuroleptic because they're available. But what I was concerned about was the exemption of two benzodiazepines if one of them was flurazepam given at night. Many people feel that flurazepam was "pushed" as a hypnotic as part of a marketing move, not because of pharmacological reasons. If you are selling chlordiazepoxide and diazepam by the millions why push flurazepam for day sedation; if it is marketed as a "marvellous hypnotic" it is in a different market. If concomitance of flurazepam with another benzodiazepine is exempted and those charts are not pulled how are the doctors going to learn by the process?

Dr. Dorsey. Well, I think it comes back to the question of what you're setting out to do. If you're setting out to eliminate bad and dangerous practice, the chances of real harm coming to somebody from taking Dalmane at night and Valium during the day are fairly remote. It's possible but not likely. If your goal in doing audit is to upgrade the standard of the average practitioner to the much, much more ambitious and much less demonstrably effective activity, then that criterion should be left in. This is precisely why we left it optional, to let the particular review organization use it according to whatever goal they had in mind. We thought that the harmful effects were not in the same league with, for example, giving an anti-psychotic drug and an anticholinergic G. I. drug at the same time.

Dr. Dennis Kussin (Montreal). We've been dealing a lot with the global kind of issue, and I would ask the panel members specifically, given the current state of our knowledge, what should the individual hospital be doing? I'm thinking of the teaching hospital where there is quite a multiplier effect if there _is_ an aberrant kind of practice in prescribing or therapy or whatever. I'm wondering, thinking of my own local hospital, what kind of things should we be doing at our local level. Should we have a committee elected by the physicians there? Should it be appointed by administrators? What kind of power should it have? What structure should the individual hospital start at this point?

Dr. Dorsey. I'll address the point briefly by saying that a lot of it again depends on what you want to accomplish. In a small to medium sized hospital with mostly private practitioners, having a committee appointed by administration is the kiss of death. Whatever the committee decides, right or wrong, will be opposed for reasons other than scientific merits. On the other hand, in a government hospital, where the whole tradition is more hierarchical in nature, then an appointed committee may make sense. So how you do it really comes down to what kind of hospital you have and what you are setting out to do. Again, I say that in terms of what's clearly demonstrable, we should get rid of the worst practice that 9 out of 10, or 95 out of 100 doctors on the staff agree is awful. It is much easier to identify it in the first place, much easier to agree on what it is, and much easier to get the kind of sanctioning that's necessary than it is to argue between a 30% staff membership who believe something should be done one way and 70% another.

Dr. Stricker. I would suggest two things, one of which is more specific than the other. First, it would be helpful for hospitals to think in terms of coalitions among local groups, because the effect of a hospital committee--working with everyone else and being a good old guy--is somewhat limited. If you could have a joint review committee within an area, so that people would move from one hospital and review in another, and if that could be done in more of an atmosphere of acceptance, I think you'd have a much better chance of people making hard decisions than if everything is done internally. The other, much less specific thing--but I think it's probably the most important of all in teaching hospitals--is if you could integrate into the training of the medical students and the training of the interns and the residents the value of review and the importance of that kind of activity. Then, rather than seeing it as something imposed out of nowhere and as another obstacle to get around, it would be an important part of their training through their initial development. I think they would be a great deal more likely to be accepting of it--accepting of it in a spirit in which it's offered, as a means to better practice--rather than seeing it as one more thing to give them trouble.

Dr. Richman. I think there are two parts to this process. Dr. Dorsey has mentioned the democratic part, where the medical staff themselves develop a committee to determine the criteria of absolutely unacceptable practice. After that point, though, there is a certain amount of autocracy necessary. If the committee has determined that there are patterns of practice that are unacceptable and if there is a practitioner who doesn't respond to those reminders, then I think it's necessary to go to the credentialling process that was mentioned this afternoon, and to invoke the process of consultation being used by that particular physician when it comes to psychopharmacology. I think that one of the problems in peer review is the familiarity of practitioners with one another; too often this is a dragged-out, continuing process, which is unfortunate. I think it's important to have the democratic part, but also, at some point, to have the consultant or the senior respected clinician involved and assisting the deviant practitioner.

Dr. Lowy. I'd like to step out of the chairman's role for a moment to join the group of panelists. There have been a number of analogies drawn throughout the day that I'd like to quibble with. One particularly is the analogy that was implied earlier, in fact by Dr. Fifer right at the beginning, of Coca Cola, the airlines, and tetracycline as examples to which we might aspire in terms of quality control. Let's take the airlines. I think what we're talking about in terms of professional quality control has less to do with the wing of the DC-10 and more to do with the skill of the pilot flying the DC-10. And in a situation where life and limb are at stake, as in flying and in medicine, we ought to be comparing our performance with the training maintenance of the efficiency and competence and the ultimate fate of pilots. Most airlines are pretty careful about this, but they also draw the distinction that Dr. Richman just alluded to, and I think it's a crucial one. Sometimes pilots are simply told that they may not fly any longer because their health is not up to it, due to eyesight, epilepsy, cardiovascular problems, fitness, etc., or sometimes their technical proficiency is so dangerous to the public that the airline, fearing law suits or feeling concern about its passengers, decides that this person can't fly. But there are a great many other instances, by far the larger set of instances, where the competence issue isn't that serious, and the person is transferred to a less complicated aircraft or is given retraining, or in some fashion is made safer. Now, hospitals probably fall into two groups here. One group is made up of those hospitals which have a group of practitioners who are not employees of the hospital or a university system, and over whom no one has direct control. They're private practitioners who are associated with the hospital where they do their work, but they're not, strictly speaking, employees of the hospital. And in those instances, obviously there's a high degree of voluntary compliance that's required before anything is done, at least at the local level. But in a great many other systems, for example all the government hospitals, most of the university hospitals, and a lot of other public hospitals, there are chiefs of staff, there are chiefs of service, there are administrative people who are mandated by somebody to exert quality control. That's been alluded to. There are a variety of mechanisms which have always been employed to try to improve the ratio between capability and danger--transferring staff, usually in face-saving fashions, encouraging a change of practice routine, occasionally retirement--so that standards can be maintained. And, only in the grossest instances is there cause for dismissal. Now, I don't know .... Perhaps the panel might comment on whether the peer review procedures we're discussing now apply to both of these circumstances, or are we really only talking about those few bad apples that were referred to earlier?

Dr. Richman. I think one of the major misapprehensions about the medical audit is that it substitutes for the clinical hierarchy or substitutes for the other supervisory mechanisms within the hospital and the medical audit is used to assess the quality of work of an individual practitioner. When that happens, it never works well. The medical audit is no substitute for the clinical hierarchy, the administrative hierarchy, or for the personnel department.

Dr. Sibley. I'd like to support that. One of my concerns is not to let medical audit kind of slide down into being a policing or punitive mechanism. I think you'll lose whatever creativity there is in a medical audit if it begins to be used that way. I would make that a clear distinction. At least in Ontario, the hospitals are operating under the Public Hospitals' Act, which clearly does identify certain lines of responsibility. For example, a head of a department can be held legally responsible for the incompetence for someone else in that department. So there are kinds of checks and balances. I'd like to mention one thing that has interested me over the last ten years, where the quality care work that I've been doing has not been in a hospital situation, but in ambulatory practices. I've gone to many practitioners and asked them privately, "Look, would you like to get involved in a strategy for you to see whether you're practicing well or not, according to some standards? Would you like to get involved in this?" We have now gone into 40 practices--all private practices in Ontario--and have never been refused the opportunity to go in and do a quality of care study in that practice. This really surprised me at first. I think there's a bit of a misconception that doctors do not want to know how well they're doing. I think they do, but they are very concerned about how that information would be used. That comes back to my first point: don't misuse the medical audit. You'll lose what creativity there is in it.

Dr. Dorsey. I have one other comment in terms of practical matters of how the hospital and the regulatory body, whatever it is--whether it's JCAH or PSRO--can interact. Often the majority of the hospital staff will, without any auditing mechanism whatever, have a good idea of who their deficient physicians are and want to do something, but lack sufficient motivation to overcome the collegial spirit or the concern of law suits, or whatever. Where the hospital wants to do it, an external regulatory body can be perceived as being ultimately responsible. For example, our PSRO was having trouble getting the hospitals in our area to comply. The federal auditors came around and told us that we had to. We told the hospitals that they had to comply or we would go under, which we had no intention of doing. That meant that some of the hospitals--the ones who knew they had, and we knew they had, problems with a particular physician--were able to say, "Now we have to go get Dr. Jones, not because we want to, but because the PSRO is on our backs, and because the federal government is on the PSRO's back". It's a way of getting people to overcome that reluctance and do what they really are largely inclined to do in any event.

Dr. Fred Grunberg (Montreal). I would just like to respond to what Dr. Dorsey said regarding the cost-effectiveness of these exercises. Is this worth a 250 million dollar business?

Dr. Dorsey. I guess part of the answer is that in the health area in the United States,$250 million vanishes without a trace. That's an accounting error. It's not something that is a major commitment, that would consume about 9% to 10% of the gross national product of the United States. I think the real question--certainly the question that is being asked rhetorically and then answered by government--is whether you are willing to put a larger share of your resources into monitoring what you're doing until you get closer to something like government and business. You may have to spend $250 million, which is big money when you're talking private dollars--it's big money in Canada and the U. S. In terms of the whole health care system, it's not much.

Dr. Sibley. I think we should be very cautious in using the cost benefit analogy. Two hundred fifty million dollars might seem to be a high cost, but to be very frank, the medical profession has never yet established its cost benefit according to what we do.

Dr. Stricker. I was reminded of something very similar by what Dr. Dorsey said. When I was in Washington once, trying to encourage them to implement the system we devised, I was speaking to Senator Stennis' legislative assistant, because he is in charge of the appropriate committee, and was saying out of naivete, "You've spent $500,000 already, why don't you do something with it?" and he looked at me and he said, "That's the amount we round off".

Dr. Albert Plante (Montreal). I'd like to know from Dr. Dorsey--whose presentation on the criteria for using psychotropic drugs was very interesting--if he knows of any such work focussing on the use of psychotropic drugs with children and adolescents?

Dr. Dorsey. The answer is that our criteria include specific subsections for children and adolescents. We also went to the American Academy of Child Psychiatry and got their comments. *(Please refer to appendix A and reference 1, p. 57 - Eds.)*

Mr. Peter Ellis (Toronto). As one of the--I think the few--non-medical or paramedical people here, I find that the presentations have been interesting. At other seminars I've attended, which have been broader-based--designed for the trustees and the administrators and the physicians--a lot of thrust has been given towards the medical-legal requirements of the trustees: insuring that they are aware that if they don't have proper auditing and appraisal techniques in place, they will be held liable. I think even here in Ontario, such a case happened in Scarborough not long ago. I don't know whether this has been deliberately not addressed today, as the thrust of the symposium was towards the medical and paramedical staff, but I would be interested in Dr. Fifer's comments as to whether this threat of liability is valid--whether, in fact, there are other influences at work that will insist that some form of appraisal is adopted.

Dr. Fifer. We didn't mean to slight trustees, I'm sure. The situation in the U. S. is similar, in that the trustees of the community hospital are legally responsible for the quality of care. Now, they have a delegation function in relation to the practitioner because they don't know good care from bad, and the practitioner has his allegiance back to the trustee internally. I guess we just didn't mention this because there aren't any trustees here, and we were talking about the technical job to be done following the delegation. But I think your point is perfectly right. By the way, the trustee is the person who has the ultimate "see to it". Let's say the medical staff doesn't do anything, or the professional staff says, "Well, we're too threatened by that to do anything about it". Ultimately, the trustee has to say, "You are going to do it, because I have that legal responsibility and must mandate its accomplishment", even if they have to theoretically change the medical staff. We could get into some interesting debates about that.

Dr. Dorsey. Particularly in private practice that is often a very difficult thing to do because the trustees cannot, in fact, change the medical staff without closing their hospital. In a rural area where there is one hospital and ten or twenty doctors, the accommodations are usually on some other basis than final mandates simply because the mandate is pretty difficult to make stick. It again comes back to what I mentioned before: it's a matter of the majority of the medical staff finally being willing, under pressure of conscience and external forces, to take the action that they believe is right. But it's very difficult for a trustee, or a board of trustees, or an administrator to mandate that a medical staff take some specific action and make it stick.

Dr. Durost. Just one comment. The last question here was concerned about the involvement of trustees, and Mr. Ellis was kind enough to say that the speakers in the panel have been talking about medical and paramedical personnel. But I think if we went back over a transcript of the day's discussion, we would find very little reference to paramedical personnel and non-physician members of treatment teams. I know that when Dr. Awad was setting up his audit here in Q.S.M.H.C., he used input from each discipline represented in the treatment team in his particular service. I would appreciate the comments from either the audience or other members of the panel with regard to the pros and cons, advantages and disadvantages, of including the broad spectrum of disciplines in review activities.

Dr. Lowy. You have to go, Dr. Stricker, so why don't you have first crack?

Dr. Stricker. This will be my parting shot because I have a plane that I'm about to miss. I think that that is absolutely essential. As a psychologist, one of the things that has always been a bone of political contention and a great difficulty is the number of situations in which psychologists and psychiatrists offer identical services--the cases where treatment does not involve medication, so that psychotherapy is involved. Identical services are offered, and yet different review mechanisms are in place. If in fact the two CHAMPUS review programs go through, what it will mean is that if a patient goes to a psychologist, he'll have one set of services which are reimbursable, and if he goes to a psychiatrist he'll have another set of services which are reimbursable. But the services are exactly the same; only the criteria are different, and that has no relevance to what the people in the office are actually doing. I think it's absolutely essential that interdisciplinary committees be involved both in the establishment of the standards and the implementation of the standards. How one goes about doing that will probably be about as easy as me getting to the airport on time.

Dr. Fifer. I want to make a comment, and it applies to something Dr. Stricker alluded to. There is now in the literature, under the name of Thomas Kiresuk, an evaluation model called a "Goal Attainment Scale Model", which is much like the model used in the CHAMPUS work. They really didn't care whether the provider of services was an M. D. psychiatrist, a psychologist, or a psychiatric social worker. As a matter of fact, they intentionally randomized the treatment-source--the practitioner--in order to get some of their studies. That comes under the generic heading of Program Evaluation, and that's an important distinction to make, conceptually. Also, Dr. Willer referred to the fact that the client had not been involved. That's wrong. Kiresuk's work had a goal set mutually by the client and the therapist, and the essence of the evaluation was evaluation by an outside observer of the attainment of that goal at various points in time--much as was mentioned by Dr. Stricker in the CHAMPUS model. Dr. Kiresuk publishes a magazine called Evaluation, of all things; it really deals with much of what you've heard today, and goes back almost ten years now. Their goal attainment scale model--Dr. Willer may wish to comment on this--has involved the client, I think, from the beginning.

Dr. Dorsey. I think that part of the question that arises is whether ultimately you're talking about a medical care system that is taking care of basically sick people and using treatment modalities like surgery, electroconvulsive therapy, and medication. In those cases most of us--not only physicians, but government as well--feel that the M.D. should finally call the shots and take the responsibility; that is very much one of the things he is being paid for, and being paid a premium, just as the airline pilot is paid a premium for flying the plane. He may get along well with the stewardesses, but when it comes time to put down the landing gear, he's the one who puts it down or doesn't put it down. We have to make the distinction between that kind of medical care and mental health services, which branch over into various kinds of helping and social services. There, maybe a team can be held responsible, or maybe people of different disciplines can. I think the other question that the insurers and government in the United States are asking is whether the latter kinds of services--the mental health services, the helping and social services--ought to be either funded or reviewed in the same way as medical care. Maybe psychotherapy, counselling, and social assistance of various kinds should be funded privately or through grants or a number of other ways, and medical services should be strictly defined as the kind that are rendered to hospitalized people with schizophrenia, manic depressive illness, or alcoholism. In that regard, there is a kind of overlap between psychologists and psychotherapy-oriented psychiatrists, whose interests and ways of doing things coincide to a considerable extent. On the other hand, biologic, largely hospital-based psychiatrists have views, practices, and use of diagnosis that are much closer to say, neurology or internal medicine than to mental health. I think this is one of the areas of continuing controversy as to how to review, and who pays, and how much.

Dr. Lowy. One of the areas we haven't gotten into today, and it's far too late in the day to begin, is the area of outcome studies related to psychotherapy. In the last decade there has been admittedly small but definite progress in this area, which at one time seemed totally impossible. Clearly, if it is difficult to establish outcome criteria for people treating hypertension or even people treating bipolar affective disorders with antidepressants or lithium, it is much more complex and difficult to look at outcome for psychotherapy. One of the promising ways of going about it is the goal attainment scaling model of Kiresuk. Surely it will not be long before we will be asked to do something like this, long before our expertise and technology permit us to say anything really worthwhile. The field, I think, is really rudimentary.

Dr. Fifer. The health services system in Minneapolis, St. Paul is an absolutely huge market, with millions and millions of dollars worth of inpatient care. Since it is now paid for by insurance, which it didn't used to be, the logical question is: "Is there any difference in the outcome if you go through an inpatient program which costs X or if you go through an outpatient program which costs Y (which is 1/20 of X), or if you go to AA for a buck a week?" People are saying "Show us that difference, because you're sending us very big bills" I believe that, always, outcome evaluations are going to be couched in terms of how much money you threw at the problem, so that if the medical model as we have characterized it is more expensive than the alternatives, the burden of proof is probably on those professionals to show that it's better.

Dr. Lowy. Of course the other problem with talk about medical or other models is the assumption that one model is likely to be useful for all the conditions we're talking about, whereas more likely different models are best suited for different things. You drew a pie this morning, Dr. Fifer, that represented the patient improving. You talked about Mr. Lalonde's booklet and you pointed out that 14% of that pie is accounted for by, shall we say, medical model activities. If you take psychotherapeutic model activities, irrespective of who delivers them, presumably they attack another, perhaps even larger portion of the pie with some overlap, but perhaps there is a considerable area with no overlap. And then if you look at various social phenomena having nothing to do with the health care system, they account for other segments of the pie. Hopefully the right model will be applied to the right segment of the pie.

Dr. Dorsey. I would just like to comment on alcoholism in particular. Most alcoholism programs are not run on the medical model, and there is even more difficulty in alcoholism than in much of the rest of the mental health field. Alcoholism has been defined as a disease, funded through health insurance, and treated in hospital by a basically antimedical approach in the majority of cases. The therapeutic community operates for $150 a day, and the physician is largely an appendage in many of these programs. The patients or clients (they are called patients on the insurance forms and clients in the program) are actively discouraged from taking any medication whatever. I think it again comes down to the two questions: the scientific question of which treatment approach or which intervention should be used for which kind of problem, and the economic question of which particular problems or which particular interventions are going to be funded out of health care dollars.

Dr. Willer. I would like to change the topic a little bit if it's okay with you. When I'm feeling really cynical about quality assurance, I reach the conclusion that it's really a bandaid for a much more serious set of problems. I was particularly impressed with the discussion about psychotropic drugs--how the group of experts decided that one set of drugs was not appropriate, and if they had their way they would ban them, but they still developed criteria for them. I'm concerned about that, and I'm not sure that quality assurance will solve that problem. It seems to me that if you look at health care--the rising costs and the concern for quality--there are three basic problems that quality assurance doesn't deal with. One is inadequate research. I don't think we know nearly enough about what works, and that's the hitch when it comes to doing quality assurance: you're going to try to establish what someone should be doing when in actual fact you don't know what that someone should be doing. The second problem is that even the little that we do know, we don't transfer to students in medical schools or residents in programs of psychiatry. I have some experience with medical schools, and what we pass on to them is probably only ten, twenty, thirty percent of what we really should; this is very inadequate education. The hospital system is not very well tuned to education, and that's a very serious problem that quality assurance doesn't address. I think the third problem is inadequate administration. The hospital system is such that it has not run itself well and I see quality assurance as a bandaid here too. Hell, even if you find somebody who is not doing the job well, you don't have a whole lot of choice to do anything about it anyway. So even if you do introduce quality assurance and even if it is a bandaid, it isn't even a good bandaid. But I just think that when I'm feeling really cynical. Do you guys have any comments on that?

Dr. Dorsey. I can comment briefly, to say that I tended to be somewhat more cynical and dissatisfied about medicine until I spent time working in business and government...... and recognized that there are very few, if any, perfect human institutions. Medicine tends to be more self-critical, I think, than either of those two large areas of human endeavor. I again come back to the point that what quality assurance can do is offer a considerable barrier to really bad quality. I don't think that it's going to affect the average very much. It'll just lop off the deviant tail and thereby affect the mean a little bit, but doing that, and doing it consistently every time, is well worth a good bit of time and effort, and is something in which the medical profession can take some pride.

Dr. Lowy. We're winding down, but I think one thing probably needs to be said. There is a basic philosophical assumption beneath the entire quality assurance discussion that we have had today and that is almost an assumption of omnipotence on the part of the health care system. The assumption is that if only we assure the best possible care and everybody practices as well as they are able to, then miracles will happen--the planes will never fall. In point of fact, medicine and all the helping professions exercise art as much as they exercise science and they always have. At some previous time in medical history, a discussion of this sort might have revolved around whether it could be established that the black bile or the phlegm or whatever humor was predominant at the time. There is no question that we are talking about the state of the art. That's the limiting factor at any given point. The state of the art is imperfect. We're talking about how to bring the level of practice, of application, up to the highest possible standard within what we know. But even that's going to fall considerably short of omnipotent expectations. So Dr. Willer's disappointment, I suspect, will continue, even if every practitioner in the health field practices up to the optimal level, because there is an awful lot that we're just not going to be able to do.

Dr. Fifer. I want to underscore the need for more research. I'm as discouraged as Dr. Willer is. We systematically say that medicine is an art and very empirical, and then we do nothing about it. Randomized control trials in our contry didn't begin until the early 50's, when we got our heads together and figured out that Isoniazid did something for tuberculosis. Since then, we've fiddled around with hypertension only in the VA system. Now RCT's are older in England, to be sure, than they are in our country, but I think it's time to excuse the medical schools from auditing. Just say, "Well, you don't have to bother with that, you're exempt from that, but get off the dime and get busy with some clinical research that begins to make some sense out of scientifically validated criteria for what works." It's embarrassing to be called on the carpet to explain the indications for taking out a child's tonsils and have the best experts say we don't know. It's equally embarrassing, I think, for a group of psychiatrists to come together and say we really don't know what the best care is in psychiatry. It's time for medical schools to begin to invest the time and effort in the controlled studies necessary to reduce some of the empiricism in medicine. We've begged off for years on this art business and I think it's a cop-out.

Dr. Dorsey. I must admit that at one point I was more impressed with research--when I was doing it actively--than now, as I've been practicing more actively recently. I'm reminded of Cervantes: "Facts are the enemy of truth". Certainly data unleavened by clinical experience can be very misleading, and I think this is one of the problems even in well-designed, well-controlled drug studies. They often get very atypical populations. For example, the ideal population in which to study any new psychotropic drug is a fairly homogenous patient population that doesn't have any other diseases. You don't take in people who have not only anxiety and neurosis, but also cardiovascular disease and liver disease. Yet, if you turn around and see where the drugs of this class are actually used, they are used widely in people whose ages are outside the range in which the original study was done, whose physical condition is different from that in which the original study was done, and whose practitioner has a very different level of expertise from that of the researcher who was doing the study. Some think that the studies are good guides, but ultimately that's part of the difference of opinion even among experts: not only what the data in a particular study show, but how those data translate to the average patient treated by the average practitioner. I think that would be arguable ad infinitum.

Dr. Thompson. I'm sitting here getting more and more uncomfortable all the time. I'm listening mostly to medical things and usually I'm accused of being too medical with my little three piece suit and all the rest. Today I find myself sitting in a very different camp. I'm sitting here thinking, "My God". I had a sense that this was the way things would go, and I suppose that's why I tried to come in today with a model that is, although somewhat confusing on its first presentation, at the same time holistic. In the centres in which I have been working for some time, most of the therapeutic contact with patients, and most of the contacts as far as diagnosis goes, are in the hands of non-medical people. The medical people have a very real role to play, and I have to question criteria that are laid on from above and from other groups of people. The more I hear, the more frightened I get that those sorts of criteria are very inappropriate at times to the work that we're actually doing. There is an interesting model at a children's centre here in Toronto--I'll name it, it's Dellcrest. It's interesting because they have taken a business management approach and said "Okay, what's a model that might work at the clinical level, that is, at the level of a child care worker dealing with a kiddie, at the level of a social worker dealing with the family, at the level of a counsellor?" What they've found is that if they go to the team and ask them, "What is it that you would really feel good about" And your patients--what would they feel really good about doing and accomplishing?" and if they ask them, "Within what times frame would you like to accomplish these things?" they find that they get some very interesting criteria sets as answers. These criteria very closely resemble those of other organizations; they're just a little bit more practical, a little bit more aligned to the work that they're doing, but not much different otherwise. The other thing they get is tremendous motivation to accomplish that which they are setting out to do. This is very close, of course, to goal attainment scaling naturally. It's old hat, except for one thing: it seems to work, and that's not old hat. I think that's different and I think it's worthwhile. They apply this at Dellcrest, as we are trying to in our agency, not just to the clinical areas, but to every aspect of the business. That's the reason for the very broad-based model--applying it to the secretaries, to the administration (which gets embarrassing at times), and applying it to everything that we do in our work at this point.

Dr. Lowy. I would like to thank the panel and the speakers from the audience for their contribution.

Finally, I call on Dr. Sibley to wind up for us.

REFERENCES

1. Brook, R. H., Quality of Care Assessment: choosing a method for peer review, N. Engl. J. Med. 288, 1323-1329, (1973).

2. Brook, R. H., Davies-Avery, A., Quality assurance mechanisms in the United States: from there to where? in: "Questions of Quality - Roads to Assurance in Medical Care", ed., Gordon McLachlan, Oxford University Press, (1976).

3. Brook, R. H., et al., Quality assurance today and tomorrow: forecast for the future. Ann. Int. Med. 85, 809, (1976).

Concluding Remarks and Conference Overview

John C. A. Sibley, M.D.

It was a privilege to be invited to participate in this conference on evaluation of quality of care in psychiatry, particularly since I am not a psychiatrist. I have, however, been interested and involved in the assessment of quality of care for some time. The organizers of this conference are to be congratulated. They have brought together distinguished individuals who have had extensive experience in the United States and Canada concerning many of the current issues in assuring a reasonable standard of quality of health care.

This volume presents the papers and ensuing discussion at the conference. The aim of the conference organizers is best served, not by attempting a review of each presentation, but rather by identifying certain themes, highlighting a few key issues, and pondering the question, "Where do we go from here?"

Why Should Psychiatrists be Concerned About the Evaluation of Quality of Care and Peer Review?

In spite of the tremendous public interest in issues of health care and, in Canada at least, increasing governmental concern with the cost and the availability of health care, physicians--and some were present at this meeting--ask, "Why should we be involved in this contentious problem of measuring quality of care and submitting to peer review?" The large number of participants in this conference indicates that psychiatrists are aware of the desire of the public and its legislative representatives for assurance that there is value received for the health care that is purchased.

The demand for public accountability is real and legitimate, and requires a thoughtful response if we are to maintain our professional integrity and autonomy. Traditionally inherent in the concept of professional responsibility is the principle of stewardship. This means that professions, in this case particularly the health professions, should behave in a manner that is consistent with publicly defined goals and needs. The public is asking increasingly perceptive questions about the quality of care received. If the professions and the institutions fail to convince the public that they are addressing issues of quality of care, public accountability of the profession will become public control. Legislative action and centralized decision making by the bureaucracy will determine what constitutes "good care". The attempts by hospitals, professional organizations, and colleges to develop procedures for ensuring quality of care should be supported by all of us.

A special study of the medical profession in Ontario, financed by the Ontario Medical Association and subsequently known as the Pickering Report (1), clearly identified the steps the profession must take to reinforce the trust and to regain the respect of the public. This survey showed that 17.8% of the public interviewed had concerns about the availability of services, 34% wanted reassurance as to competence, and 46% identified the need for good human relations if trust were to be restored. Fortunately, professionals are becoming active in these areas in Canada. Dr. Henry Durost presented a useful historical account of these developments and described the progress in establishing clinical care evaluation programs in provincial psychiatric facilities in Ontario. The number of psychiatrists, other health professionals, and institutions involved in medical audit and peer review activities is impressive.

The Major Purpose of Quality of Care Evaluation

There are many issues contained within the term "quality assurance". These range from patient satisfaction to technical care and outcome studies. Without denying the importance of utilization studies and related aspects of cost control, we should clearly distinguish activities that focus on cost containment from those that focus on quality. Health planning, health economics, and public policy are important issues. For the practising psychiatrist in Ontario, however, it is more important to assess, through a variety of strategies, the appropriateness, usefulness, or efficacy of his or her decision making.

As one reviews the papers in this volume, one is impressed by the research being done by many of our colleagues from the United States. This conference was the richer for their contributions. A word of caution, however, may be in order. There are significant differences between our two countries, not only culturally and politically, but also in the funding and delivery of health care. There is only one third party in the health care system in Canada--the government. This ensures that the public has reasonable access to health care; there is uniformity in the provision of health care; and it is universally applied. However, our health care system does have problems of insensitivity, inability to fine-tune and correct problems such as poor distribution of health professionals. There are also difficulties with centralized and cumbersome authority.

Presently, in Ontario at least, the problems of utilization and cost containment are being met by what can best be described as a policy of rationing health care. A recent Ontario Economic Council Report (2) showed that the total health expenditure for Canada as a percentage of the GNP was 7.1 in 1970 and still 7.1 in 1976; the comparable figures for the United States were 7.2 in 1970 and 8.9 in 1977. The current quality assurance issue in Ontario is: Can we develop a system which will measure the quality of care, identify its strengths and weaknesses, ensure corrective feedback, and respond to it with sensitivity? Furthermore, can this be done in such a manner that the public and its legislative arm can have reasonable confidence in the process? This is a tall order.

Factors in the Development of Quality of Care Assessment

It is clear from the papers presented that there is no simple or single strategy yet developed which can measure, in either absolute or relative terms, the quality of care. Dr. Fifer referred to Brooks' (3) excellent article in which he reviewed the state of the art and identified priorities for further research in the quality of care. Brooks pointed out that quality assessment involves two basic concepts; the quality of technical care and the art of care. Technical care refers to the various diagnostic and therapeutic maneuvers undertaken in the delivery of health care. The art of care refers to the style, manner, sensitivity, availability, communication skills and, in general, the behavior of the provider. Positive art of care, hopefully, should encourage certain behaviors of the patient, such as increasing compliance, improving health habits, and the responsible use of medical services. Psychiatrists, I am sure, are particularly concerned with this component of quality of care. We are increasingly preoccupied with behaviorally induced illnesses from misuse of drugs or alcohol, cigarette smoking, accidents, and stressful life styles. We know very little about measuring the efficacy or the efficiency of intervention in this area of the art of care, and a great deal of research must be done. Strategies need to be developed, tested, and validated before large-scale interventions and programs are instituted. Possibly, this is a lesson we can learn from the PSRO experience south of the border.

Another issue that needs to be addressed is the relative usefulness of process and outcome studies. Current medical audit and peer review activities are primarily process measures; they attempt to record and measure what physicians or psychiatrists do. Process studies are based on the assumption that certain activities of the physician affect the patient's outcome.

These studies have some advantages. It is relatively easy to identify, from observation or from medical records, what physicians do. Studies can be carried out over a short period of time and they are relatively inexpensive. The major disadvantage, of course, is that we do not know how directly many process activities relate to specific outcomes. Sackett et al. (4), in a well-designed, randomized control clinical trial, have clearly demonstrated that an extensive patient health education program did not improve patient compliance in taking medication.

Understandably, there is a great effort to develop outcome measures to assess quality of care. Outcome measurement is logical and theoretically reflects the ultimate goal of therapy. A disadvantage is that many factors other than the process of medical care may be potent determinants of outcome. As Brooks (3) points out, extensive research in the major disabilities is required in order to identify specific relationships between process and outcome. If these relationships can be determined, quality assessment programs will take a tremendous step forward because process items can be recorded and measured with relative ease.

Dr. Richman and Dr. Durost stressed the appropriate use of medical audit and peer review and thoughtfully introduced a word of caution by identifying the limitations of such studies. For a medical audit to influence physician behavior it should be current and focussed on specific topics; it should identify problems and recommend specific corrective action. There must be prompt feedback and discussion with the physician, team, or unit involved. It should be a positive educational endeavour rather than a punitive procedure. It must also be a continuing process. Because of the methodological limitations of peer review, it cannot be equated to quality of care. Measuring physician behavior is useful and encouraging change in behavior is admirable, but until we know more about the relationship of physician behavior, or process, to outcome, we cannot equate medical audit or peer review with quality of care.

Measuring quality of care in a hospital setting is difficult enough. Assessing it in ambulatory settings is even more difficult. As Dr. Kerr White has indicated, out of a population of 1,000 at risk, 720 visited a physician, 100 were admitted to a community hospital, and 10 were admitted to a university or a reference hospital per year. If we are to go where the action is, we must develop strategies for assessing physician competency in the ambulatory setting. If these figures hold true for patients with emotional and psychiatric disorders, it is clear that an approach such as that described by Dr. Stricker for a peer review of outpatient or ambulatory psychological services is highly relevant and extraordinarily important. Similarly, Dr. Dorsey's study on the prescribing of psychoactive drugs might be particularly important in an ambulatory care setting. There is evidence (5) that how well physicians prescribe drugs may reflect how well they handle a variety of indicator conditions.

Given the complexity of the problems facing us in attempting to establish quality of care appraisal systems, are there criteria we can use in developing such systems? Dr. Durost quoted Tugwell's criteria: a system should be reproducible, have outcome validation, clinical credibility, accuracy, comprehensiveness, sensitivity, a scoring index for measurement, and, finally, should be feasible and able to be introduced at reasonable costs. There are no easy shortcuts and we should be cautious in accepting substitutes.

In our concern to ensure physician competency we are, at times, in danger of assuming that we can substitute knowledge for competence. While we cannot provide competent care without reasonable knowledge, we can be very knowledgeable and yet not behave in a clinically competent manner. Legislation has been introduced in a number of States requiring attendance for a specified number of hours at continuing medical education programs. Even if it can be assumed that attendance at such programs increases knowledge, it does not follow that the increase in knowledge changes physician behavior. I am not aware of any well-designed, methodologically sound and validated study that shows a strong correlation between continuing medical education and improved professional behavior, let alone improvement in patient outcome. Extensive continuing medical education programs in themselves will not solve the problem of quality of care. When we can point to knowledge deficits as a key factor in inadequate care, then we must educate as specifically and as promptly as possible.

Where do we go from Here?

Simply because we do not have all the answers in quality assessment does not mean that we should stand still. While searching for improved strategies we must judiciously use the best approaches that are available. There is good evidence that peer review and medical audit can change physician behavior even though in many cases we do not know whether it directly affects patient outcome. The participation of physicians to be audited in the construction of an audit may be an even more important factor in changing behavior than the conduct of the audit itself.

It is clear that research into the issues of quality of care is urgently required. Funding must be available. Basic and applied research are still necessary, but only if we follow through with health care research can we get answers to such questions as the efficacy and efficiency of diagnostic and therapeutic interventions, and finally achieve quality assurance. This requires the full support of the professions, institutions, funding agencies, and the government.

Dr. Awad and his colleagues, Dr. Durost and Dr. McCormick, are to be commended and congratulated on their initiative in holding this conference on the evaluation of quality of care and peer review in psychiatry. The papers presented here have identified the issues, reported on progress, and described promising new strategies. I am sure that all those attending the conference would join me in expressing the hope that this will lead to a second conference at which the results of further research in quality assessment can be presented. Results of carefully designed studies can be shared; our understanding of quality of care strategies can be improved; and we can move closer to our goal of developing a system of quality assurance and thereby discharging our public accountability.

Dr. Anne Somers, addressing a Conference on Assessing Physician Performance in Ambulatory Care (6), referred to the need for physician involvement in quality assessment. She stated that the concept might be likened to the "categorical imperative" propounded some 200 years ago by Immanuel Kant:

> At a time when philosophers were hotly debating the existence of God and the relevance of competing ethical principles, Kant concluded that, while His existence could not be proved, it behooved the individual to conduct himself "als ob" or"as if" the universe were ordered in accordance with a universally binding moral law.

While we continue to question and research, we must also continue to behave as if audit, peer review, and other quality assessment strategies lead to quality of care and quality assurance, even though at this point it has not been proven. We have a great deal of work to do, and even with our present state of knowledge we must act as though there is a categorical imperative.

REFERENCES

1. Pickering, Edward A., Report of the Special Study regarding the Medical Profession in Ontario, prepared for the Ontario Medical Association, (1973).

2. Barber, M. L., Evans, R. G., Stoddart, G. L., Ontario Economic Council Occasional Paper #10: Controlling Health Care Costs by Direct Charges to Patients: Share or Delusion?

3. Brook, R. H., et al, "Quality Assurance Today and Tomorrow: Forecast for the Future", Annals of Internal Medicine, 85: 809,(1976).

4. Sackett, D. L., et al, "A Randomized Clinical Trial of Strategies for Improving Medical Compliance in Primary Hypertension", Lancet, 1: 1205-1208, (1975).

5. Sibley, J. C., et al, "Quality of Care Appraisal in Primary Care: A Quantitative Method", Annals of Internal Medicine, 83: 46-52, (1975).

6. Somers, Anne, "Public Accountability and Quality Protection in Ambulatory Care", Conference Proceedings: Assessing Physician Performance in Ambulatory Care. The American Society of Internal Medicine, San Francisco, Calif., June 1976.

Index

Accountability (*see Public Accountability*)
Accreditation Council for Psychiatric Facilities 44
Accreditation Surveyors 22
Achong, M.R. et al 15, 16, 17
Adverse developments 54
American Psychiatric Association,
  development of screening criteria 51
  psychopharmacological screening criteria 57-74
American Psychological Association 82
Anderson, O.W. 48, 91, 94
Assessment methods, faults in 6
Audit (*see Medical audit*)
Awad, A.G. 44, 48, 77-79

Barber, E.A. 118
Brook, R.H. 11,45,47,97,100,112, 116, 118
Calne, R. 79
Canadian Council on Hospital Accreditation 41
Canadian Medical Association, patient care appraisal 45
Canadian Psychiatric Association, Task Force on Peer Review 45
Carden, T.S. 11
Carstairs, G.M. 31
Chart review 42
CHAMPUS 81
  regulations for group therapy, individual psychotherapy,
    marital therapy 86
  patient's participation 86
  third party payers 81, 82
Civilian Health and Medical Program for the Uniform Services (*see CHAMPUS*)
Claiborn, W.L. et al 89
Clinical policies and procedures 22
Clinical record 21, 22, 25
Confidentiality, third party payers 88
Consumer Report 3
Continuing medical education 6,7,117
Coran, M.J. et al 89
Cost containment (*see Quality assurance, cost*)
Cost crisis 9
Cowan, E. 16
Credentialing 6, 8
Criteria 3, 4
  input 3
  outcome 4
  process 4

DiMascio, A. 79
Disability payments 13
Documentation 24
  requirement, for 22
  psychiatry's response to requirement, for 26
Donabedian, A. 11
Dorken, H. et al 89
Dorsey, R. 49-76
Drug prescribing practices, deficiencies 77,78
DuMas, F.M. 92, 93, 95
Durost, H.B. 41-48

Education, postgraduate 78
Eliot, T.S. 28
Evaluation of medical care
  criterion-referenced 3
  norm-referenced 3

Fifer, W.R. 1-12
Firth, J. 47, 48

Garfinkel, P.E. 78, 79
Goal Attainment Scale 106
Goldberg, W.M. 13-17
Gottlieb, R.M. et al 79
Greenberg, R. A. et al 11

Havelkova, M. 39
Hawthorne effect 15
Health expenditure, Canada 115
Health Professional Educational
  Assistance Act 7
Hill-Burton legislation 7
Hospital
  accountability 9
  functional units 14

Illness behavior 13, 14
In-depth patient care review 37
Involuntary patient, freedom to
  choose treatment 50

Jakobs, C.M. et al 30
Joint Commission on Accreditation of
  Hospitals (JCAH) 2, 41

Kahn-Hut, R. 30
Kent, I. et al 47, 48
Kiresuk, T. 106, 107

Langley, D.G. 48
Lantham,P.M. 3l
Lee/Jones Report 2
Lee, R.I. et al 11

Malpractice crisis 10
McAuliffe, W.E. 11
Medicaid 8, 9, 50
  mills 10, 27
Medical audit 6, 22
  committees 42

Medical care evaluation, semantics 4
Medical education, peer review 16
Medical schools 8, 77, 110
Medicare 8, 9, 50
Menninger, R.W. 30, 82, 89
Mental health care, models
  medical 91
  non-medical 92
  antimedical 92, 93
Mental state examination 53
Metarazzo, J.D. 90
Meyer, A. 19, 30
Murray, J. A. 43, 48

National Institute of Mental
  Health 51, 56
Nicoll, S.W. 29, 30
Nork Case 15

Outcome, quality of care assessment 116

Patient care appraisal
  Canada-U.S. differences 46
  characteristics 42, 43
  problems 45, 46
    medicolegal aspects 46
    methodology 45
    validation 45
Patient education 116
Patient participation 88, 94, 107
Pecarchik, R. et al 95
Peer review
  outpatient psychological servi-
    ces 81-90
  shortcomings 2
  use of psychotropic drugs 49-57
Pickering, E.A. 118
Pickering Report 114
Pirsig, R. M. I, II
Polypharmacy 54
Postgraduate training 16, 78
Professional care evaluation 42
Professional credentialing 8
Professional involvement,
  alternatives to 9
Professional Standards Review
  Organizations (PSRO) 45, 81
Psychiatric Audit Team Seminars
  (PATS) 44
Psychiatric diagnosis, peer review
  84, 85, 86
Psychiatry's response to self-assess-
  ment 26

Psychopharmacological screening
criteria
antianxiety medications 58, 59
antiparkinsonism medications 60,61
antipsychotic medications 61-66
applications in Canada and U.S. 56
fixed-ratio combinations
products 66-68
inpatient documentation 57
lithium 69-71
monoamine oxidase inhibitors 74
outpatient documentation 58
philosophy 52
psychostimulant medications for
children 71, 72
purpose 52
tricyclic anti-depressants 72,73
Psychopharmacology, deficiency in
training 78
Psychotropic drugs 49
Public accountability 2,8, 9, 113

Quality
assessment 4
control 1, 2, 4, 5, 15, 94
crisis 10
definition 1, 23
discussions 2
measurement 3
purpose 93
Quality assurance 4, 6, 9, 19, 23,
26, 28
accrediting agencies 26
Canadian perspective 93
conflicting process 91
cost containment 91, 94
definition 23, 28
difficulties in application to
psychiatry 27-29
locus 7
problems 6
reluctance of professionals 10
Quality of care evaluation
consumer satisfaction 2
cost-effectiveness 104
factors in development 115
purpose 114
role of government 8

Randomized control trials 110
Richman, A. 19-31
Riedel, D.C. et al 30
Room, R. 30

Sackett, D.L. et al 118
Sanazaro, P.J. 30
Screening criteria, application in
Canada and U.S. 56
Select Committee on Psychiatric
Care Evaluation (SCOPCE) 82
Shader, R.I. 79
Shapiro, A.K. et al 31
Sibley, J.C. 113-119
Somers, A. 118, 119
Standardized treatment programs 27
Standards, health professional
role 8
Stricker, G. 81-90
Swanson, A.L. 48

Thermostat, control model 5
Thompson, M.G.G. 33-39, 48
Tissue Committee 15, 42, 46
Trustees, medical-legal requirements
105
Tucker, G.J. et al 30
Tugwell, P. 45, 48

Undergraduate training, quality
control 16

Venn diagram 35

West End Creche Child and Family
Clinic 33
Willer, B. 91-95